American National Red Cross Text-Book
On First Aid And Relief Columns A Manual Of Instruction How To Prevent Accidents And What To Do For Injuries And Emergencies

Charles Lynch

Alpha Editions

This Edition Published in 2021

ISBN: 9789354445781

Design and Setting By
Alpha Editions
www.alphaedis.com
Email – info@alphaedis.com

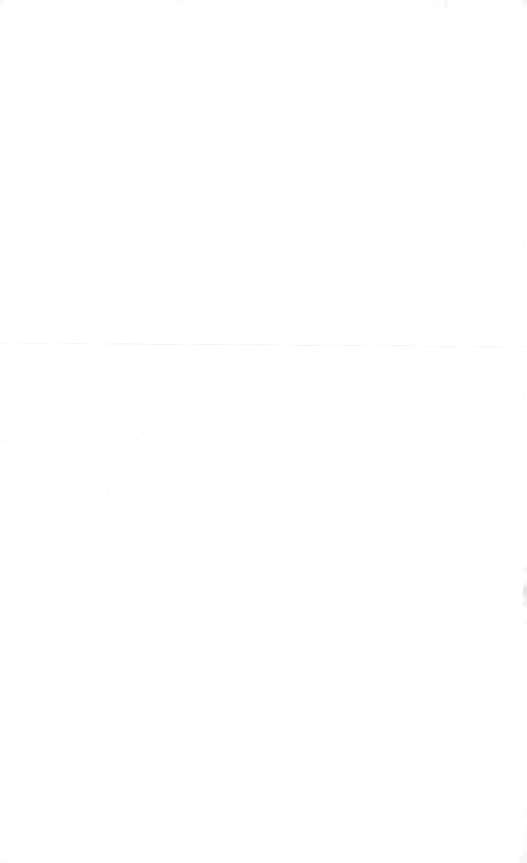

PREFACE

This small manual on the subjects of First Aid and Relief Columns represents an important departure so far as books of this character are concerned. Notwithstanding the many excellent works already in existence on first aid instruction, none of the writers, so far as I know, has given much thought to teaching the prevention of accidents. While this subject is necessarily treated rather briefly here, at least enough is said to call attention to the importance of prevention as contrasted with cure, and for this reason it seems to me peculiarly appropriate that this book should have the indorsement of the Red Cross, as the beneficent mission of that association, like that of the good physician in treating disease, should be to go deeply into causes which are responsible for the physical sufferings of humanity rather than to resort solely to palliative measures.

Another novelty in the present manual is that it treats not only of first aid as given by the individual, but also of relief columns, bodies designed to administer first aid as organizations. Army conditions emphasize the necessity for the creation of organizations in order that first aid may be given with maximum efficiency, and there are many situations in civil life, such as vast concourses of people, great fires, railroad disasters, etc., which equally demand first aid organizations instead of individuals who, however well taught they may be, must, under such circumstances, work at cross purposes unless they are united into a disciplined body in which the special duties of each are carefully defined.

In view of these facts, it is believed that this book will serve to fill a place of its own in the ever-increasing movement for the relief of human suffering.

R. M. O'REILLY,
Brigadier General, Surgeon-General. U. S. Army.

CONTENTS

AMERICAN NATIONAL RED CROSS TEXT-BOOK ON FIRST AID AND RELIEF COLUMNS.

CHAPTER I.

ANATOMY AND PHYSIOLOGY.

A workman, in order that he may repair his machine, must know exactly how it is made and how it operates. This is exactly the knowledge which a surgeon should have of the human body. The latter is such an extremely complicated mechanism, however, that months and years are needed to acquire such knowledge. Fortunately, it is not necessary for the first-aid student to go so deeply into these subjects. His efforts to relieve suffering will, and should without more knowledge, be confined to emergency treatment. To render this intelligently it is necessary to know comparatively little of anatomy and physiology or, in simpler language, of the structure and mechanics of the human body.

In this chapter will be found all facts on these two subjects which are essential for the student of first aid. But even the comparatively simple anatomy which he must know cannot be learned from books alone. What is said here should, therefore, be added to by careful study of the skeleton, and of the form of its more important bones and of his own body or, better, that of a comrade. Thus the positions and relations of the more important structures may be clearly pictured in his mind. Good charts may also be made of considerable assistance to him. The services of a competent teacher, while perhaps not indispensable, must always prove of great value.

The subjects of this chapter and those of the next two, while essential, are very dry and difficult for the beginner, and it is suggested that the student be not required to memorize them at first, but that he run rather hurriedly over them, returning to them again and again in connection with practical work in caring for supposed accident and emergency cases.

THE BODY.

The body is composed of hard and soft parts. The bones are the hard parts and the muscles and the internal organs, such as the heart, lungs, liver, etc., constitute the soft parts.

BONES.

The bones are hard and firm and together make up the Skeleton. **The skeleton**—

Forms a strong and rigid frame-work for the body.

Supports and carries the soft parts.

Protects vital organs from injury.

Gives attachment to muscles.

Forms joints so that movements are possible.

The skeleton is divided into three parts:

1. **The Head,** made up of the Cranium, a bony case which encloses and protects the brain; and the Face, with the eyes, ears, nose and mouth. The only movable bone in the head is the lower jaw.

2. **The Trunk,** which is divided into two parts by a muscular partition—the diaphram. The upper portion is the Chest, which contains the esophagus or gullet, the lungs, the heart and some large blood-vessels. The lower portion is the Abdomen, in which are found the stomach, liver, kidneys, bladder, the intestines and other organs.

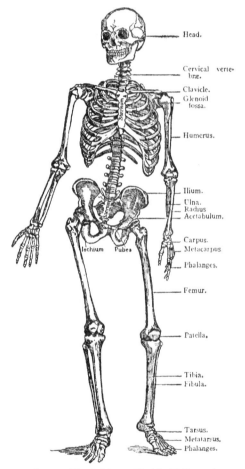

FIG. 1.—-The skeleton. (*Gould's Dictionary.*)

The trunk is formed of several bones which are of interest to the first-aid student.

The Spinal Column, a strong pillar with several curves, is made up of a number of bones called vertebræ with a softer substance called cartilage between them. At its lower end, the spinal column terminates in the broad Sacrum or Rump Bone and the pointed Coccyx. The spinal column is hollow and contains the spinal cord, a continuation of the nervous substance of the brain. The spinal column supports the head and the ribs, and is itself supported on the pelvis.

The Ribs, 12 in number, form the greater part of the walls of the chest. All the ribs are connected to the spinal column behind, but the two lower ones on each side are shorter than the others and are not connected to anything in front. The 10 upper ones on each side are united to the Breast bone.

The Breast-bone or Sternum is a flat, dagger-shaped bone which forms the front of the chest. Above it forms joints with the Collar-bones, being notched for the purpose on each side.

The Pelvis is a wide, strong, bony basin formed of the Haunch bones (ilia) at the front and sides and partly behind where it is closed by the sacrum and coccyx. It supports the trunk and forms joints with the lower limbs.

3. **The Extremities Comprise the 2 Upper and the 2 Lower Limbs.** Each upper limb is made up of the Scapula or Shoulder-blade, a flat, triangular bone at the back of the shoulder; the Clavicle or Collar-bone, a curved long bone placed horizontally across the upper part of the chest above the first rib; the Humerus, the bone of the upper arm; the Radius and the Ulna, the two bones of the forearm; and the Hand, which has 8 small, irregular bones in the Carpus or wrist, five Metacarpal Bones for the hand itself, and 14 bones in the fingers and thumb.

Each lower limb is made up of the Femur or Thigh-bone; the Patella or Knee-cap; the Tibia and Fibula, the two leg bones; and the Foot. The foot is made up of the Tarsus, the heel, and part of the ankle; the instep with seven irregular bones; 5 Metatarsal Bones for the middle of the foot; and the toes with 14 bones.

The principal interest which bones have for the student of first aid is that they may be broken or fractured, one of the commonest accidents. (See Fractures, page 65.)

TEETH.

The teeth appear in two crops; the first or milk-teeth, 10 in each jaw; the second or permanent teeth, 16 in each jaw. The milk-teeth usually begin to appear from 4th to the 7th month after birth, and in the 6th year the first of the permanent teeth begin to replace them. This process goes on for from 6 to 7 years until all the teeth are permanent, though the wisdom-teeth do not appear until from the 17th to the 21st year. The milk-teeth, when they are being replaced by the permanent teeth, become loose so that they may be easily pulled. The permanent teeth are closely anchored to the jaw, however, and both strength and skill are required to pull them.

The teeth are covered with a very hard substance called enamel. This is pierced by decay so that the nerves are exposed and are liable to become inflamed and very sensitive and painful, which is the cause of toothache.

JOINTS.

Wherever two or more bones are in contact or touch each other they form a joint. The ends of bones forming a joint are covered with a smooth substance called cartilage or gristle, so that they may move without friction on each other. Joints are hermetically closed by a flexible sac, the capsule, which secretes an oily fluid. This fluid lubricates a joint just as oil does an engine. The ligaments of a joint are strong, fibrous bands which may themselves form the capsule or may be separate from it. The most important joints to study are the hip and shoulder, which are ball-and-socket joints having movements in all directions as well as rotary movements, and the elbow, wrist, knee and ankle, hinge joints. These have only to and fro movement like an ordinary hinge.

Joints are of importance to the student, as bones are liable to be put out of place or dislocated at the joints. (See Dislocations, page 62.)

MUSCLES.

The movements of bones at the joints are effected by the Muscles.

The muscles, the flesh or meat, form two-fifths of the body by weight. They are made up of red fibres which have the power of shortening or contracting, so that if one end of a muscle is fixed and the muscle is contracted the other end will pull on and move whatever it is attached to. By doing this muscles cause all the movements of the body. For example, the biceps, the big muscle at the front of the upper arm, by contracting causes the elbow joint to bend by bringing the forearm closer to the upper arm. All muscles are somewhat on the stretch, as otherwise prompt movement would be impossible. Some of the muscles are attached to bones by Tendons or sinews. These are strong, fibrous cords. They may be well seen in the wrist.

Muscles are of two classes: Voluntary muscles, such as those of the arm and leg—these are under the control of the will; and Involuntary muscles, such as the heart—these work independently of the will. By this wise provision of Nature all vital processes go on without our being compelled to give any thought to them.

Voluntary muscles are of prime interest both in fractures and in dislocations, as their pulling causes displacements and their resistance offers the chief obstacle to setting fractures and to reducing dislocations. (See Fractures and Dislocations, pages 62 and 65.)

CIRCULATION

The Heart.—In order that the blood may reach all parts of the body it is, of course, necessary that some force shall propel it. This is provided by the Heart, which is not the seat of the feelings, but a most skillfully devised pumping machine.

The heart is about the size of a man's fist and is located in the chest between the lungs. It is a hollow, muscular organ, with valves which close and prevent the blood from flowing backward, all its force being expended to send the blood forward. The beat of the heart which we feel in the chest is its contraction by which it is made smaller inside, thus forcing the blood to the furthest parts of the body. After the heart contracts it dilates or becomes larger inside and the valves open so that it may fill with blood. The next contraction again forces the blood forward, and so on as long as a person is alive.

The heart contracts usually about 72 times per minute.

While, as has just been stated, the heart is a pump, it is not a single but a double pump, being divided into two entirely separate halves by a muscular partition. The left side of the heart, or the left pump, drives the blood through the body, and the right side drives it through the lungs alone.

Blood-vessels.—A series of closed tubes, or blood-vessels, as they are called, carry the circulating blood. They are of three classes: 1, Arteries; 2, Capillaries, and 3, Veins.

1. **Arteries.**—Leaving the left side of the heart is the largest artery of the body—the Aorta. This strong tube is just about large enough so that a man's thumb may be introduced into it if

it is separated from the heart. It soon divides into branches which again branch and rebranch, the individual branches constantly growing smaller in size, to reach finally the furthest parts of the body. It should be remembered, too, that the smaller branches of the arteries join freely with one another. The blood passes from the heart to the aorta and thence to the smaller arteries, not in a steady stream but in waves, each of which is produced by a contraction of the heart. The beat of these waves causes the Pulse, which may be felt not only at the wrist and temple, but also anywhere else an artery is near enough the surface of the body. Naturally, if an artery is cut, there will not be a steady stream flowing from it, but the blood will be expelled in spurts or jets. The walls of arteries, especially those of large calibre, tend to remain apart when divided.

As the course of the blood in the arteries is away from the heart toward the extremities and the head, if an artery is cut, in order to stop the bleeding the artery must be compressed either on the side of the heart or on the bleeding point itself. Pressure on the further side of the cut will, as may be easily understood, do no good so far as stopping bleeding from an artery is concerned. It is also necessary to press on the artery on the near or heart side as close to the bleeding point as possible. This is because arteries in their branching and re-branching join each other, and if pressure is made on an artery far above the bleeding point, so many branches may bring blood into it between the point of pressure and the bleeding point that a great deal of blood will be lost, notwithstanding the fact that the main branch is blocked by pressure at a distant point. However, it is not in every part of the body that arteries lie near enough to the surface to be compressed in their course. Moreover, it is necessary in compressing an artery to select a point where a nearby bone gives a hard surface to press against. Therefore, the student of first aid must know, first, the situation and course of the principal arteries and, second, the points on which to exert pressure.

Without going into details, the aorta may be said to have three great branches which are of particular interest to the student of first aid. One of these, the Carotid, supplies the head and neck with blood; the second, the Subclavian, the upper extremity; and the third, the Femoral, the lower extremity.

The table which follows gives certain necessary information regarding these arteries and their branches.

Artery	Course	Point on which to exert pressure.
HEAD AND NECK.		
Carotid	From upper, outer edge of breast bone to angle of jaw.	Deep. Down and back, an inch to the outer side of Adam's apple.
Facial (a branch of carotid).	Diagonally across the lower jaw from below upward.	On the face, an inch in front of the angle of the lower jaw.
Temporal (a branch of carotid).	Upward one-half inch in front of ear.	On skull, immediately in front of upper part of ear or on temple.
UPPER EXTREMITY.		
Subclavian.	Across the middle of first rib to arm pit.	Deep. Down and back over centre of collar-bone on first rib. Shoulder should be drawn down first.
Brachial (a branch of a branch of the subclavian).	Descends along inner side of biceps muscle. About line of seam of coat.	Against humerus by grasping and pulling biceps to outer side.

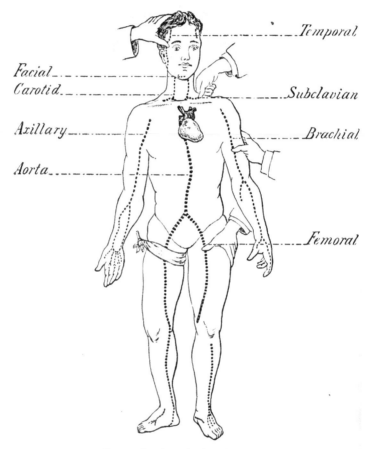

FIG. 2.—Arteries and points of pressure.

Artery	Course	Point on which to exert pressure.
	LOWER EXTREMITY.	
Femoral.	Down thigh from pelvis to knee, line from middle of line between point of hip and centre of pelvis in front to inner side of knee.	Against femur high up inner side in line given about three inches below upper end of line.

Arterial bleeding is always most serious, because blood thrown out in jets from the cut artery with each contraction of the heart is rapidly lost. The blood which spurts from an artery is always bright red in color, as arterial blood has not yet lost the characteristic bright red of the oxygenated blood from the lungs.

2. **Capillaries.**—The arteries, as they go further and further from the heart, become very small and thin-walled, till they finally terminate in still smaller vessels which are called capillaries, from the Latin word meaning a hair. The capillaries form a delicate net-work of vessels everywhere, and give the rosy color to the skin. Slight pressure on the skin will cause a white spot to appear. This is because the pressure has forced the blood from the net-work of capillaries and the white skin is seen instead of the rosy color due to the presence of the blood in the capillaries. In capillaries the pulse, or contraction wave from the heart, is no longer apparent, as these fine, hair-like tubes break up the waves. Slight cuts or pricks of the skin are sufficient to divide some capillaries and therefore to cause bleeding. Naturally, on account of the minute size of these vessels, bleeding from them, except from a very large surface, is not dangerous to life. Capillaries branch so freely that pressure used to check capillary bleeding, to be effective, must be made on the bleeding point. The blood lost

from capillaries is no longer bright red in color like that from arteries, but is somewhat darker.

3. **Veins.**—The blood-vessels which return the blood to the heart from the points furthest from it are called veins. They may be easily recognized as the blue lines under the skin. Everywhere many capillaries unite to form minute veins, these unite to form larger veins, and finally these vessels become very large before entering the right side of the heart. The best known of the large veins is probably the jugular vein of the neck. Bleeding from a cut vein is in a continuous flow instead of in jets, as is the case with bleeding from arteries, and it is mainly through this difference that one distinguishes venous from arterial hemorrhage. Venous blood, too, is dark, bluish-red in color, as the oxygen in the blood stream is lost in its passage through the capillaries. While bleeding from veins has not the almost terrifying appearance of arterial bleeding, a dangerous amount of blood may be lost from a large vein. As the course of the blood in the veins is toward the heart, in stopping bleeding from them pressure must never be made on the side toward the heart.

The Blood.—The Blood is a fluid which carries properly prepared food, oxygen, and heat to nourish and warm all parts of the body, from which it also removes waste materials for final expulsion. These processes go on constantly as long as life lasts. Coagulation is the property of the blood which is of most interest to the student of first aid. While the blood is circulating in the living vessels it remains fluid, but as soon as this influence is removed it coagulates or clots, thus tending to stop bleeding. It is easy to see if Nature did not provide this safeguard that the slightest scratch sufficient to draw blood would result in the loss of all the blood in the body. The rate of loss would be regulated simply by the size of the opening just as is that of water flowing from a pipe. Very rarely a person is found whose blood does not clot. These people are called "bleeders," and they often bleed to death from a trivial injury, such as the pulling of a tooth.

In order that one may know what to do to stop bleeding, it is necessary to know what conditions favor or impede coagulation of the blood. First in importance, in order that blood may clot, is comparative rest. A spouting stream of blood will never clot except where it falls and is therefore at rest. Free exposure to air also favors clotting. Coagulation is likewise more promptly effected by contact with foreign substances, especially if they afford many points on which clots may form. Gauze is a good example of such a material. Cobwebs are also, and they were much used even by surgeons before the danger of dirt in a wound was so well understood.

For further discussion of this subject, see Wounds and Hemorrhage, page 78.

RESPIRATORY SYSTEM.

The Respiratory System consists of the Nose and Mouth, the Windpipe and the Lungs. All of these organs except the lungs may be regarded simply as the passageway for the air going to and coming from the lungs. Naturally, anything which blocks this air in its course will interfere with the supply of air to the lungs and complete blockage will result in early death from smothering or asphyxiation.

At the upper end of the windpipe is the Larynx, part of which we know as the prominent Adam's Apple in the throat. As the larynx is in front and the gullet is behind, food passing to the latter must pass over the upper end of the larynx and would naturally enter it if some protection were not provided. This is afforded by the epiglottis, a muscular flap or curtain which falls into position, covering the upper end of the larynx so that ordinarily food does not enter it. Sometimes, however, the epiglottis does not do this, especially if one swallows quickly or attempts to talk while swallowing. In this case choking results from food entering the larynx, or, in common words, one has swallowed the wrong way. The attempt to give food or water to an unconscious person will also result in choking him because his epiglottis does not close.

The Lungs may be described as two soft, spongy structures, each of which is bag-like in shape and is made up of air cells with many blood-vessels surrounding them. The lungs are hermetically enclosed in the chest, so that when the cavity of the chest is increased or diminished in size, the same effect is produced on the lungs themselves. Certain muscles are of great importance in filling and emptying the chest and lungs. Ordinarily, the muscular movement consists simply of the bellows action of the chest and the up and down movement of the diaphragm. In order that the chest may be enlarged to its greatest capacity, however, some of the muscles of the upper extremity must also take part. In order that they may do so, the arms are raised vertically above the head, so that certain muscles attached to the chest wall and to the upper extremities will, when the latter are fixed, raise the ribs and thus enlarge the chest. The chest, too, is elastic and direct pressure upon it will diminish its size and so force the air from the lungs. (See Artificial Respiration, page 164.)

The rate of respiration is 16 per minute.

The function of the lungs is to aerate or oxygenate the blood. The small blood-vessels surrounding the air cells which the pure air breathed in finally reaches, carry dark blood which has lost its oxygen in the tissues. This blood receives oxygen from the pure air and returns to the heart as bright arterial blood. The air which is expired from the lungs has not only lost its oxygen to the blood, but has also received certain impurities from the latter.

DIGESTIVE SYSTEM.

This is the system by which the food is received and is prepared for the use of the body. From the mouth the food enters the esophagus or gullet, through which it passes to the stomach and then to the small and large intestines from which the residue is expelled. In its course it is acted on by the various digestive fluids, which change it so that it may be absorbed into the blood. The two largest glands in connection with the digestive system are the liver and the pancreas, the former supplying bile and the latter pancreatic juice. Both of which are digestive fluids.

A part of the intestine, and near the junction of the small and large intestines, is the Vermiform Appendix, which is so liable to inflammation with the resulting disease called Appendicitis. The appendix lies at some distance under the wall of the abdomen, at a point on a line from the prominent point of the hip-bone in front to the navel, about one and one-half inches from the former.

The abdomen is lined with a delicate membrane called the Peritoneum, which secretes a fluid and so permits smooth movements of the various movable organs which it contains. This membrane has no communication with the interior of the abdominal organs, and when, through an injury or disease, their contents enter it, or a foreign body enters it from outside, it becomes inflamed and Peritonitis results.

It is also necessary to remember here that absorption of anything swallowed and thus introduced into the stomach is very rapid, so that if this material is of a harmful nature it must be promptly expelled if bad consequences are to be avoided.

NERVOUS SYSTEM.

Through the Nervous System the actions and functions of the various parts of the body are performed, regulated and controlled. This system is really a double one. One part is composed of the

Brain and Spinal Cord and the Nerves connected with them, and the other is the so-called Sympathetic Nervous System.

The Brain is the seat of the will, intellect, voluntary motion, and sensation. From it come the nerves of the special senses, which include smell, taste, sight and hearing.

The Spinal Cord is a continuation of the brain, and gives off many pairs of nerves in its course through the spinal column.

The Nerves are white cords which originate in the brain, pass into the spinal cord and finally emerge from it, then ultimately break up and become very small, reaching all parts of the body, much as do the blood-vessels. The nerves carry nervous impulses from the brain which govern the movements of the voluntary muscles as well as convey sensations to the cord and finally to the brain.

The nervous system has been aptly compared to a telegraph system, the brain being the central office in which the messages originate and to which they come from outside, and the nerves, which really constitute a great cable made up of many nerves in the cord, being the wires which carry the messages to and fro.

Pressure on the brain from any injury, on account of pressure on the nerve centres is likely to result in loss of movement, of feeling or speech, and often in total unconsciousness. Severe injuries of the cord from destruction of nerves cause paralysis below the injury. Naturally, high injuries are most dangerous, and destruction of the cord immediately below the brain results in instant death. Division of a nerve anywhere in its course will result in loss of motion or feeling below, depending on whether the nerve carries a message from or to the brain.

The Sympathetic Nervous System.—This system is called the involuntary nervous system, as it operates independently of the will. Through it, the bodily functions necessary for life—circulation, respiration, secretion and excretion—are carried on, sleeping or waking, without conscious effort. The sympathetic nervous system consists of two cords which are placed on either side of the spinal column. These have numerous swellings, or ganglia, as they are called, and send many small nerves to the organs, such as the heart, blood-vessels, lungs, etc., which are not subject to the control of the will. Perhaps the action of the sympathetic nervous system is best illustrated by the effect which is produced by a hard blow on the abdomen. Such a blow often paralyzes the great sympathetic ganglia here, which, in consequence, cease to main-

tain the contraction of the blood-vessels and they dilate so much that a great part of the blood in the body can enter them, so the injured man will become unconscious because of the small amount of blood furnished to the brain.

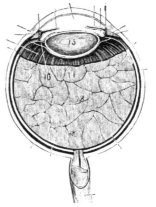

Fig. 3.—The eye. (*Potter's Anatomy.*)

SPECIAL SENSES.

It is hardly necessary to discuss the special senses here. Some of the organs of special sense are, however, subject to injuries peculiar to themselves, and therefore it is important to know something of their anatomy.

The Eye is the organ of sight. It is a ball surrounded by three coats. The internal, the Retina, is an expansion of the Optic Nerve, which enters the eye-ball at the rear. At the front of the eye is the Iris with an opening in its centre, the Pupil. Just back of the iris is the Lens, which focuses rays of light just as does any other lens. Back of the lens, filling the whole eye, is trans-

parent matter called the Humors of the eye. Covering the eye-ball
in front is a delicate membrane called the Conjunctiva. Protection to this membrane is afforded by the Eye-lids when they are
closed, but when they are open it is very liable to injury and to the
entrance of foreign bodies. These are commonly spoken of as

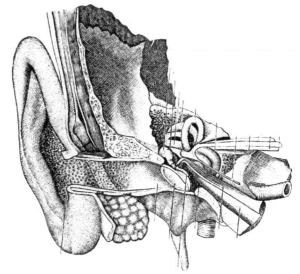

FIG. 4.—The ear. (*Gould's Dictionary.*)

"something in the eye." On account of the sensitiveness of the
conjunctiva, they cause much pain and distress. The eye-ball
itself is well protected from injury, as it is situated deeply in the
head and the brows overhang it. Pointed objects may, however,
enter it. When this occurs severe damage almost always results.

The Ear is the organ of hearing. That portion of the ear which we see is called the Pinna. Leading from it is a passageway called the Auditory Canal, which is separated from the middle and the internal ear by the Ear-drum. The auditory canal is not quite straight, and it is important to know that it may be straightened by pulling the pinna backward and upward.

Rupture of the drum is a very serious accident which is caused by a loud concussion near the ear or by putting objects, especially pointed ones, into the auditory canal, as well as by disease.

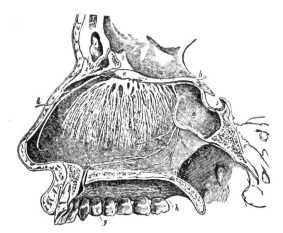

Fig. 5.—The nose. (*Potter's Anatomy.*)

The Nose.—The sense of smell is located in the upper part of the nose, which is separated from the mouth by the hard and soft palates. Both mouth and nose open into the Pharynx behind. The nose is well supplied with delicate blood-vessels, which are easily broken, with resulting nose-bleed.

SKIN AND MUCOUS MEMBRANE.

The skin affords the covering for the entire body. Under it is a fatty layer, the padding, which assists it to prevent the escape of the body heat which is produced by chemical processes in the interior of the body.

One of the most important functions of the skin is to act as a defense against the introduction of germs into the tissues of the body. Germs cannot pass through the unbroken skin, and any injury which is accompanied by a break in the skin makes a breach in this defense and is therefore much more serious.

At all points where openings occur in the surface of the body, such as the mouth, nose, etc., the character of the covering changes as soon as it becomes internal instead of external. Take the cavity of the mouth, for example, it is easy to see that its lining is much thinner and more delicate than the skin. This is characteristic of the covering of all such cavities, which is called the Mucous Membrane. While poisons are not absorbed through the skin at all, absorption through mucous membranes is more or less rapid.

CHAPTER II.

GERMS OR MICROORGANISMS.

INFLAMMATION.

While the body may rightly be regarded as a machine, it is subject to one class of injuries to which other machines are not liable. The injuries referred to are caused by microorganisms, or germs.

Of recent years so much has been written on the subject of germs that it might be thought that everybody should know all about them. This is by no means the case, however, and it is probable that on no one subject are erroneous ideas more commonly held. This is not the place to discuss the germs or microorganisms which are responsible for contagious diseases, but only those which are of importance so far as wounds are concerned. By far the commonest and most important of these are the so-called pus germs, which are very small organisms—too small to be seen except through a powerful microscope. These germs cause inflammation and the formation of pus, or matter. They exist in countless millions, but they do not live in the tissues of our bodies and must, therefore, always enter them from outside. This is a most important fact to remember. It is also important to know that pus germs do not float in the air and so cannot be carried to a wound from the air. Pus germs are found on the surface of our bodies, on knives and other objects which cause wounds, in the dust of houses, in water, etc., and also on surgical instruments and dressings unless special means have been taken to free them of germs or, in other words, unless they have been disinfected. Surgically clean means simply free of germs.

Suppose a wound is received, what happens? If pus germs do not gain access to it, there will be no inflammation and it will heal quickly and kindly; but if, on the other hand, the wound is infected by pus germs, this means that inflammation will follow, more or less matter will form, and there will be some absorption of poisonous products from the wound which may result in the more severe forms of blood-poisoning and almost inevitable death. But as pus germs are so generally present, it may appear that under ordinary conditions they would always be carried into a wound when it is received, either from the surface of the body or by the object which causes the wound. This is true, but if only a few pus germs are carried into the tissues they will dispose of the germs without trouble and no harm will result; moreover, unless too many pus germs are carried into the body, the blood resulting from the injury will often wash so many out that the tissues can dispose of the few left with little difficulty. This is exactly the reason why a wound which bleeds freely is less likely to prove dangerous afterward. With the ordinary wound, therefore, we can never be sure immediately after it has been received whether or not pus germs are present in it in sufficient numbers to infect it and our duty is quite clear. We must assume that the wound is not contaminated and must use every care not to contaminate it by our hands, by instruments, dressings, etc. This is best accomplished by covering it with a disinfected dressing, as this will prevent contaminated articles from coming in contact with it. (See Compresses, page 42.) But if no such dressing is available, it is best, when possible, to leave it exposed to the air, for, as has been stated, little danger of contamination is to be feared from the air. Ordinary water is dangerous, as it may contain many pus germs.

This liability to infection not only exists at the time a wound is inflicted, but afterward so long as the wound is raw. Every precaution to prevent infection should, therefore, be observed during all this time.

The symptoms of inflammation in a wound are heat, redness, pain, swelling and partial or complete loss of use of the wounded part. The severity of these symptoms varies considerably with the virulence of the germs which enter the wound—for they are by no means equally virulent—and with the depth of the wound. We hear occasionally of a person who has received a slight scratch having a very severe inflammation of the injured part, and perhaps dying from blood-poisoning. In such a case we may be very sure that the pus germs which entered the trivial wound were very virulent. Usually, however, the course of such wounds is not severe. The pus germs which enter it at the time it is received. or afterward, cause some irritation. This brings more blood-cells to the part and we have inflammation. Some of these cells are destroyed by poisonous products of the pus germs. This gives rise to the formation of pus, but the blood-cells form a barrier against the germs and they cannot advance further. A scab made up of blood, pus and some dirt forms on top of the wound, helping to protect it from further infection, and healing takes place under the scab, which is gradually pushed off by the healing tissue. Most of us have had numerous opportunities to follow the course of such wounds in slight injuries to our hands.

Suppose the infected wound is deep, however, exactly the same process takes place usually, but it is carried much further, and instead of the moderate inflammation with a small amount of pus which is produced before the blood-cells form their barrier, inflammation is severe, a large amount of pus forms and an abscess is produced. The original wound has probably closed by this time, so this abscess is surrounded on all sides by the inflamed tissues of the body. Its contents are irritating, and unless it is very small will not be absorbed, so it works toward the surface, causing inflammation meanwhile. As soon as the contents escape, however, the irritation is removed and the sides fall together and healing takes place.

With virulent infections, especially deep ones, as the microorganisms breed much more rapidly in captivity, the poison of the pus germs is so powerful that the blood-cells cannot form a barrier, the inflammation spreads, and the poison gains entrance to the blood-vessels and is carried to the brain, the heart, etc., and death is very likely to follow from blood-poisoning. The symptoms of this condition need not be mentioned here, but it is well to remember that it is not the immediate result of an injury, but appears only after what has been described above has taken place. Usually some days are required, but the period is shortened in a very virulent infection.

In plain words, therefore, the infection of a wound means more pain, slower recovery, perhaps a scar which will give trouble afterward and a certain amount of danger to life; and deep wounds are more to be feared than superficial ones. There are, of course, proper methods for the treatment of infected wounds, but these will not be discussed, as they do not fall under the head of first aid.

Tetanus, or Lock-jaw, is caused in the same way as pus infection. That is to say, a wound is infected with the germ of tetanus, absorption from it takes place, and the result is lock-jaw. The special germ of tetanus does not exist in all localities, but where it does even more care, if possible, should be exercised so far as wounds are concerned.

Rabies should also be mentioned here; it will be discussed at length under the proper heading.

CHAPTER III.

FIRST AID MATERIALS.

Bandages; Compresses; Plaster, Collodion and Similar
Substances; Splints; Tourniquets; Heat; Cold;
Stimulants; Emetics.

It is almost as important for the workman responsible for the operation of a machine to know how to make practical use of the tools which he requires to repair it as to know how the machine is constructed and how it operates. This is equally true for the first-aid student. Therefore, this chapter is devoted to his tools and repair materials.

BANDAGES.

Bandages are used for the following purposes:

To keep dressings in place.
To fix splints.
To stop bleeding by pressure.
As slings.

Whatever the bandage used, care must be taken that it is not put on too tightly. It should be firm and secure, but must not be so tight that it presses and constricts at any point, for this will interfere with the circulation by cutting off the blood supply, and if the bandage is left in place for some time even so severe an injury as mortification or actual death of the part may be caused.

Any bandage may be fastened by a knot or be pinned or sewed. If a pin is used, a safety-pin is preferred, as it holds better and one

25

is less likely to be scratched by it than by the pin with unprotected point.

The reef knot, as it is secure, should always be employed in place of the granny knot. To tie the reef knot proceed as follows: Hold the ends of the bandage in the two hands; wind the end held

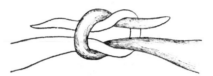

Fig. 6.—Reef knot. (*Davis.*)

in the right hand over that held in the left; then wind the end now held in the left over that held in the right and bring it through the loop. When a choice is given, the knot should be placed where it causes no discomfort to the patient and where it may be easily reached.

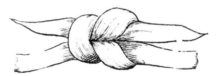

Fig. 7.—Reef knot. (*Davis.*)

The kinds of bandages used are:

The triangular or Esmarch bandage.

The roller bandage.

Special bandages.

Triangular Bandage.—The triangular bandage is perhaps most suited for general first-aid work, as it can be easily made, is not difficult to apply as a temporary dressing and is not likely to be put on so tightly that it will cause injury by stopping the circulation.

The triangular bandage is preferably made from unbleached cotton cloth, though any strong cloth will answer. Bed sheets,

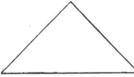

FIG. 8.—Triangular bandage.

pillow cases, napkins and handkerchiefs are all used in case of emergency. It is desirable that the piece of cloth for the bandage be not less than 34 to 38 inches square. It is folded diagonally and is cut across in the fold; of course, this will give two triangular bandages. While made triangular bandages may be readily bought, the only advantage they possess is that most of them have illustrations showing methods of application stamped upon them.

The triangular bandage may be applied in three ways:

      Unfolded
      Folded, broad
      Folded, narrow.

Unfolded means that the bandage is used in the form of the whole triangle.

To fold, broad, the point of the triangle is brought to the middle of the opposite side, and then the bandage is folded into two, lengthwise.

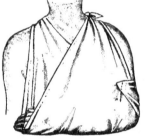

FIG. 9.—Brachio-cervical triangle.
(*Esmarch and Kowalzig.*)

To fold, narrow, the same method is adopted, but three instead of two lengthwise folds are made.

It is, of course, necessary to determine in each case of injury in what special way the triangular bandage will be used and persons expert in its use are very skillful in adapting it to special cases. Certain set methods have, however, been found by experience to be the most generally useful, and these will now be described.

The most important uses of the unfolded triangular bandage are the following:

1. **Arm sling.**

Place one end of bandage over shoulder of uninjured side. Allow length of bandage to hang down in front of chest so that point of triangle will be behind elbow of injured arm. Bend elbow of injured arm to a right angle. This will bring forearm across middle of bandage. Then carry lower end of the bandage over the shoulder of the injured side and tie to the upper end behind the neck. Bring the point of the bandage at the elbow forward to the front and pin there so that bandage is snug but does not pull. (Fig. 9.)

This makes an excellent arm sling, but even without a bandage a good sling may be made for the arm by pinning the sleeve or the skirt of the coat to the front of the coat. (Fig. 12.)

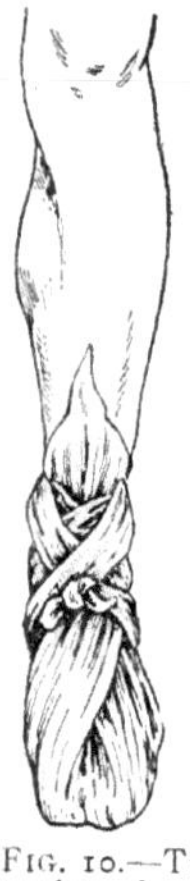

2. **Foot bandage.**

Fig. 10.—Triangular bandage for foot.

Spread out bandage. Place foot in centre with toes toward point. Raise point over toes to instep in front. Bring both ends forward, cross them over instep and tie them round the ankle. (Fig. 10.)

This bandage has but a limited range of usefulness.

3. **Hand Bandage.**

This is applied exactly like the foot bandage. The bandage is spread out. The hand is placed on it, palm down, with the fingers toward the point (if desired, the hand may be closed), and the wrist is at the long side. The point is then brought over the back of the hand to the back of the wrist and the two ends are crossed over the wrist and tied.

This bandage will be found useful more often than the preceding one.

4. Head Bandage.

First, fold a hem about one and one-half inches wide at the long side of the unfolded triangular bandage. Place the bandage so that the hem lies squarely across the forehead just above the eyes

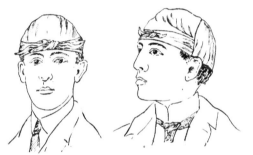

Fig. 11.—Triangular bandage applied to head.

and the bandage is over the head with the point hanging down the back. Carry the two ends around the head above the ears, cross at the back and tie them across the forehead. Draw the point down tight, turn it up and pin it at the top of the head with a safety-pin. (Fig. 11.)

This is a useful bandage.

The best example of the use of the triangular bandage, Folded Broad, is the following:

1. The Broad Arm Sling.

First, fold the bandage broad. Place one end over the shoulder of the uninjured side and allow the other end to hang down in front. Bend the forearm of the injured side to the required height, bring the hanging end under it and in front of it and over the shoulder of the injured side and tie the two ends behind the neck.

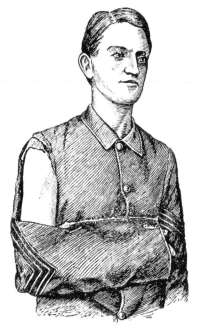

Fig. 12.—Arm sling made from patient's coat sleeve.
(*Drill Regulations H. C., U. S. A.*)

The triangular bandage, Folded Narrow, is sometimes called the cravat bandage, and in practice by folding, the cravat is made wider or narrower as required. As may readily be seen, a cravat may be made of use in any part of the body. It is especially useful to hold splints, dressings, etc., in place and to check bleeding when applied snugly so as to compress the bleeding point.

The following are good examples of the use of the narrow triangular bandage, or cravat.

1. **Eye Bandage.**

Place the centre of the cravat over the injured eye, bring the ends to the back of the head and tie. (Fig. 13.)

2. **Jaw Bandage.**

For this, two cravats are necessary. Apply the centre of the first square across the chin in front, bring the ends to the back of the neck and tie. Place the centre of the second cravat under the chin, cross the ends over the top of the head, bring them down and tie under the chin.

3. **Neck Bandage.**

The centre of the cravat is placed over the injured place and the ends are carried around the neck and tied as convenient. This bandage may sometimes be improved by the use of

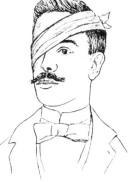

FIG. 13.—Eye bandage.

a cardboard support which is held firmly in place between the layers of the bandage.

4. **Bandage for Palm of Hand.**

Place the centre of the cravat on the palm of the hand, cross the ends at the back of the hand and again at the front of the wrist and tie at the back of the wrist. (Fig. 14.)

The cravat may also be used for an arm sling. It is applied in exactly the same manner as the triangular bandage folded broad. When the cravat is used to hold splints or dressings in place on an extremity it is simply carried around the splint, or dressing, and the limb, and is tied at the most suitable point. Of course, the number of cravats employed for this purpose is dependent on the size of the special splint or dressing.

The Roller Bandage.—The roller bandage may be used for any of the purposes already described, though as sometimes employed by the surgeon it is rather too complicated for the student of first aid. Lengths cut from the roller bandage may, of course, be always used to replace the narrow triangular bandage, and for the unskilled this method of application is always to be preferred to that usually employed by the surgeon, which consists of

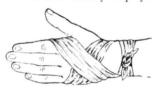

winding the roller around and around the part which it is desired to cover. This method of application makes the roller bandage especially valuable in maintaining pressure so as to stop capillary bleeding, to fix dressings after operation, etc. These are not,

FIG. 14.—Cravat for palm of hand.

however, questions which often confront a student of first aid, so if they were the only ones the use of the roller bandage might be wholly disregarded here. But this is not the case. The first-aid student should know how to take advantage of any appliances he may have at hand and he is very likely in an accident to find it much more convenient to obtain the roller bandage which may be found in every drug store, and for this reason he should know the principles of its application.

Roller bandages are usually made of muslin, cotton cloth, flannel, gauze or cheese cloth, and they may be improvised by tearing strips from a sheet and rolling them up. By far the best material is gauze or cheese cloth. This is elastic and adapts itself well to the part to be bandaged so that it is easy to apply and does not have the disadvantages of the old inelastic bandages of muslin, etc., which in unskilled hands are very apt either to be pulled so tight on one edge that they cut off the circulation or to be so loose that they will not stay in place.

While roller bandages may usually be readily bought, it is well to know how they should be rolled. One end of the bandage should be turned over for a distance of about 6 inches, this lap should be folded on itself and this process should be repeated till a small hard roll is formed. Then place the bandage on the thigh (the foot should be on a stool or chair so that the thigh is nearly at right angles to the body) with roll of bandage near the body,

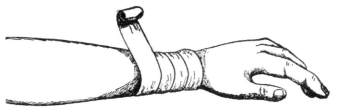

FIG. 15.—The circular. (*Davis.*)

length of bandage at bottom of roll and bandage extending down the thigh. Roll, beginning with the fingers of right hand running down to the wrist, and repeat till bandage is completely rolled. The left hand is used to hold the bandage tight and even. The bandage when completed should be in a hard roll with even edges. It may be fastened with a couple of pins.

Roller bandages are preferably used in the following sizes:

For the finger, $\frac{3}{4}$ of an inch wide and 1 yard long.

For the arm and head, $2\frac{1}{2}$ inches wide and 4 to 6 yards long.

For the leg and thigh, 3 inches wide and 6 to 8 yards long.

For the chest and abdomen, 4 to 5 inches wide and 8 to 12 yards long.

3

The bandage 2½ inches wide and 4 to 6 yards long is the most generally useful.

While it is not, of course, absolutely necessary to use the bandage best adapted in size for the part to which it is to be applied, it should be remembered that it is very difficult to bandage satisfactorily a small part with a wide bandage. Any bandage when rolled may

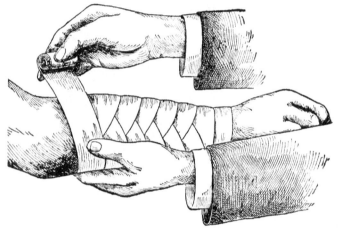

FIG. 16.—The reverse. Preparing to reverse. (*Davis.*)

be easily cut through with a sharp knife and thus a bandage of the required size may always be obtained.

The roller bandage is applied by holding the roll in the right hand, the loose end being in the left and laying the outer side of the end on the place where it is desired to start the bandage.

The simplest method of application is the Circular, but this can be used only when the part to be bandaged is of nearly the same circumference throughout. This is the case with the forearm above the wrist and with the fingers. Moreover, in first-aid work the roller bandage is usually applied to hold splints or dressings in place which much extends the field of the circular method of application as, especially with splints, an even circumference is likely to be presented. The circular method is also more often available with gauze bandages for on account of their elasticity they adapt themselves to slight pulling much better than do bandages made

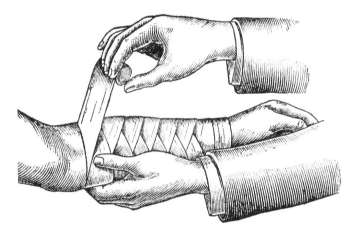

FIG. 17.—The reverse. The roller reversed. (*Davis.*)

of stiffer cloth. The circular method of application consists simply of a series of circular turns from below upward, each turn overlapping the upper third of the one below.

Where the part is larger at one end than the other, at the start a few turns should be made round and round one over the other, then begin to move up the limb, using the circular method as long as a turn overlaps the preceding one about one third. It will be found as soon as the limb increases notably in size that if the bandage lies flat, spaces will be left. To prevent these spaces, the Reverse must be employed. The Reverse is generally considered to be the most difficult point to learn in the application of the roller bandage. This is not quite the case, however. While it is certainly much more difficult to bandage successfully a part larger at one end than the other this is due rather to the fact that one not experienced in bandaging is likely to try to force the bandage instead of at once resorting to the method which allows it to lie flat, and thus to make unsightly and insecure loops at the back where they are not immediately seen than to any real difficulty in making the reverse itself. Bad bandaging in this as well as in other respects can only be avoided by practice and care.

To make the Reverse, place the thumb of the left hand on the lower edge of the bandage to hold it in place, slacken the bandage between the hands (about 3 inches) and turn the roller one half over toward you. Pass the roller under the limb keeping the lower edge of the bandage parallel with that of the turn below, reverse again at the proper point and so on. The reverses should be made so they lie in the center of the limb or to its outer side and all reverses should be in one line up the limb.

The figure-of-8 bandage is found specially useful about joints. It consists of a series of loops each overlapping the one below by about two-thirds the width of the bandage. The middle part is over the bend of the joint while the loops lie one below the other above it. (Fig. 18.)

The spica bandage is a modification of the figure-8 bandage, having one loop much larger than the other.

Precaution.

In addition to those already mentioned, some other precautions must be observed in the application of the roller bandage:

Always bandage from below upward and always bandage from within outward, over the front of a limb.

Always bandage firmly, but never too tightly or loosely, and use firm, equal pressure throughout the bandage.

Always in bandaging a limb, leave the tips of the fingers or of the toes uncovered so that they may be seen. If the tips of the fingers or toes become blue and cold or if great pain is complained of it is

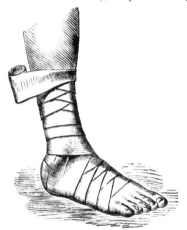

FIG. 18.—Figure-of-8 of foot. (*Heath.*)

almost certain that the bandage has cut off the circulation and it must be loosened or dangerous results may follow.

Never reverse the bandage over a sharp bone and always use the figure of 8 over a joint.

Always place the part to be bandaged in the position in which it is intended to leave it, as otherwise change of position may result in cutting off the circulation by drawing the bandage too tight at some point.

Never put on a bandage under, but always over a splint.

Always in applying a bandage immediately after an injury remember that there may be swelling and use care in order that the bandage may not become too tight from this cause; always be ready to remove or to loosen a bandage when such swelling makes it too tight.

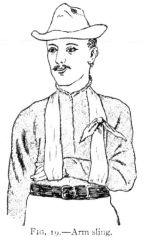

Never apply a bandage wet, for as it dries it will shrink and become too tight.

A very valuable exercise in the application of the roller bandage is afforded in bandaging the leg from the foot to include the hip. This gives an opportunity to practice all the methods of application which have been described.

The fact that lengths cut from the roller bandage prove useful in the hands of those unskilled in bandaging has already been mentioned. There are, however, three special bandages made in this way

FIG. 19.—Arm sling.

which are so simple and well suited to their special purposes that they should be known to anyone interested in bandaging.

1. **The Arm Sling** will be first described. For this a 3 or 4-inch roller bandage is required, preferably the latter. Bend the forearm on the arm at the angle at which it is desired to hold it, this is usually about a right angle. Put the end of the roller about midway between the forearm and shoulder and hold for a moment to get length required when it may be allowed to drop. But before doing so pass roller in front and under forearm just in front of the

elbow. Then carry roller along front of chest to the shoulder on the injured side, over this shoulder to back of neck, in front of sound shoulder, down to make loop for hand, back over sound shoulder, back of neck and in front of shoulder of injured side to starting point where length required will be cut off and the ends will be tied together. Two loops have, of course, been made, one for the forearm near the elbow and the other for the hand.

2. **The Four-tailed Bandage** is the second of these bandages. This is especially useful for fractures of the lower jaw and for injuries of the head. The four-inch roller bandage is wide enough to make it for the former. It should be folded lengthwise in the centre and cut or torn in the fold so as to leave 2 or 3 inches in the middle of the bandage which in applying the bandage is placed over the chin. The lower ends are then carried up over the top of the head and tied there while the upper tails carried back are tied at the back of the neck. For injuries of the top of the head the four-tailed bandage made in this way from the four-inch roller bandage will usually be

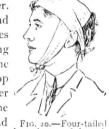

FIG. 20.—Four-tailed bandage of head. (*Stewart.*)

found too narrow. It may, however, sometimes be used especially if more space is left in the middle or it may be made from two lengths of the four-inch roller by sewing or even by pinning them together with safety pins for the required distance in the middle. When available, a piece of cloth from 6 to 8 inches wide, and 3 feet long should be used for this bandage. To apply it the middle of the bandage is placed on the top of the head, the two front ends are carried back and tied at the back of the neck and the two rear ends are carried forward and tied under the chin.

3. **The T Bandage** is the last of these bandages which demands our attention. It is used only for the crotch, especially to hold

dressings on that part of the body. It is made from two lengths of a 3-inch roller bandage. To the centre of one of these 1½ yards long is sewed or pinned at right angles the other which is 1 yard

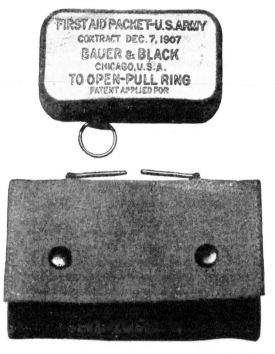

Fig. 21.—Metal case and canvas pouch, United States Army first-aid packet.

long. The bandage is applied by placing the long strip around the waist with the short one at the middle of the back. The long strip is then pinned in front and the short strip is brought forward between the legs to join the long one at the centre in front where it is pinned.

Special Bandages.—The only special bandage which need be mentioned here is the one supplied in the first-aid packet of the

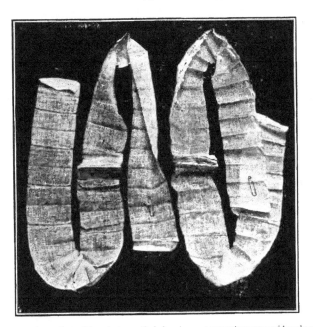

Fig. 22.—Army first-aid packet unrolled showing compress in centre of bandage.

United States Army. In each of these packets are found two long gauze bandages with compresses of gauze sewn to them in the centre. While these bandages are intended primarily for bullet wounds, as such wounds are those most commonly met with in war, they are useful for other purposes. The directions of the army in reference to the application of this bandage to wounds are, in part, as follows:

1. If there is one wound, carefully remove the paper from one of the two packages without unfolding compress or bandage and hold by grasping the outside folds between the thumb and fingers.

2. When ready to dress wound open compress by pulling on the two side folds of bandage, being careful not to touch the inside of the compress with the fingers or anything else.

Still holding one roll of the bandage in each hand, apply the compress to the wound and wrap the ends of the bandage around the limb or part until near the ends, then the ends may be tied together or fastened with safety-pins. The second compress may be applied over the first or may, if the arm is wounded, be used for a sling.

If there are two wounds opposite each other, use one compress opened out, but with the folded bandage on the back, for one wound; and hold it in place by the bandage of the compress used to cover the other wound.

3. If there are two wounds not opposite each other, apply a compress to each.

4. Be careful not to touch the wound with your fingers nor handle it in any way, for the dirt on your hands is harmful and you must disturb a wound as little as possible. The bandaging will stop ordinary bleeding.

The actual application of this bandage to a wound is even more simple than the directions indicate.

COMPRESSES.

Compresses have already been spoken of in connection with the army first-aid packet. A compress is simply something which is used to press on or, in other words, to cover an open wound. It should always be sufficient in size to do so with a lap of at least one and one-half inches on all sides. Compresses should preferably be made of gauze or cheese cloth.

Above everything else they should be safe to apply to wounds. That is to say, they must have been properly disinfected in the first place, and in the second they must not be contaminated by the fingers or anything else in the handling necessary to apply them. (See chapter on Germs or Microorganisms.) This is the great advantage of the army first-aid packet which is so prepared by the manufacturers that it is safe to put in direct contact with a wound and is then protected from accidental contamination by being enclosed in a sealed metal box. Moreover, the compress is so attached to its bandage that only gross carelessness in applying it will contaminate it then. A number of other first-aid packets are manufactured which contain compresses that may be safely applied to a wound, though none is quite so easy to handle without accidental contamination as the Army packet. Each has printed directions on the box or container which must be carefully followed, If a first-aid packet can be procured it should always be used in preference to anything else to dress a wound. The next choice should be sterile or antiseptic gauze. Small packages of such gauze suitable for compresses may be bought in most drug stores. (Sterile gauze is ordinary gauze in which the germs have been destroyed by heat and antiseptic gauze is ordinary gauze in which germs have been destroyed by an antiseptic, usually bichloride of mercury.) In a city, therefore, one may easily procure a safe compress and all he need do is to handle it so that he will not contaminate it. This may be accomplished by holding it not with the fingers, but by the paper which covers it, allowing only the inner surface of this paper to come in contact with the gauze and never removing part of the paper until it has served this purpose. If, by chance, the gauze is touched by the hand great care should be taken

to drop the untouched part on the wound and to place the gauze
which has come in contact with the hand as near the outer layer of
the dressing as possible.

As already mentioned under the heading Germs or Microorganisms, unless a safe gauze can be procured it is much safer to leave a
wound exposed to the air than to cover it, but this will not always
prove practicable. It is especially in localities where there are no
drug stores in which gauze can be bought that circumstances
render it necessary to cover wounds. In such localities it may be
hours before the services of a doctor can be procured, so an uncovered wound will be exposed for a long time to accidental contamination which will be almost inevitable from the hands or clothing of
the patient who must perhaps be moved. A compress, too, affords
an excellent means of checking bleeding, being often all that is
required for this purpose. Under such circumstances, therefore, it
will be necessary to make a compress which, if not as safe as is
desirable, is, at least, as good as can be procured. First, as surgically clean cloth for the compress as can be obtained should be
used. This will be found in a towel, a handkerchief or other cloth
of the same kind which has recently been laundered and has not
been used since it was washed. Preferably, this cloth should be
boiled for 10 minutes or soaked in a solution of 1–1000 bichloride of
mercury, corrosive sublimate, for an equal length of time. (Tablets of corrosive sublimate are in common use; they are known
as antiseptic tablets. This substance is a deadly poison and its
solution cannot be made in metal vessels.) The process recommended will give a compress which is safe to use, but an important
practical difficulty is presented in applying such a compress to a
wound. It will, of course be so wet that it will not be possible to put
it on the wound without squeezing some of the water out of it. To
do this the compress must necessarily be handled and, as already
explained, pus germs exist in countless millions on the hands. If

possible, therefore, the hands must be cleaned surgically, which means they should be freed of germs. This should be done by active scrubbing for 5 minutes with hot water, soap and a nail-brush, paying special attention to the nails. Preferably the hands should be washed under a tap instead of in a basin, and if a basin is used the water had best be changed two or three times. As a further precaution, when corrosive sublimate is procurable, the hands after being washed should be soaked in a 1–1000 solution of that chemical for a period of 5 minutes. The hands must not be wiped and they must not touch anything except the compress. The piece of cloth which is intended for a compress may now be taken from the vessel in which it has been boiled or disinfected, but in so doing the operator should be very careful not to allow his hands to come in contact with that part of the compress which he intends to put on the wound. On the contrary, he should pick up the piece of cloth by its outer surface and, holding it at all times by this, squeeze the water from it until it is comparatively dry and then put it on the wound without delay. If a fairly large piece is taken for the compress and if previous to boiling it is folded so as to fit the wound it will be handled much more easily and safely.

When no facilities are available for washing and disinfecting the hands, naturally this must be omitted, but the same precautions should be taken in handling the compress. Suppose, however, that in addition the compress cannot be boiled or disinfected, and yet it is absolutely necessary to have one. In this case one should again take a towel, handkerchief, etc., which has just been laundered, and without unnecessary handling apply its inner surface to the wound. Towels, handkerchiefs, etc., which have been used or handled, though they may look clean, are never so in the surgical sense and are therefore particularly dangerous to use as compresses.

No attempt should be made to wash or to disinfect a wound. These are matters for the surgeon, and for him only under favor-

able surroundings and conditions. It is as unjustifiable for a
student of first aid to wash or to attempt to disinfect a wound as
it would be to probe it. If he leaves the wound undisturbed and
untouched except with the safest compress that can be procured, he
will have done his best and the patient should be immeasurably his
debtor. While if he goes further than this he may be solely responsible for much unnecessary suffering and perhaps even for an unnecessary death.

PLASTER, COLLODION AND SIMILAR SUBSTANCES.

These, of course, seal wounds on which they are used, so that if
any pus germs have been introduced they are in the most favorable
condition for doing harm. The use of plaster (except court
plaster, to cover a trivial scrape not involving the entire thickness of
the skin) must be absolutely condemned, for not only does plaster
seal the wound, but it is also very likely not to be surgically clean.

Collodion and similar substances are, of course, extensively
used on wounds, and the popular idea seems to be that they actually form a skin which protects the wound. This works very well
if the wound has not been contaminated by the wounding agent, or
subsequently before the collodion is applied. On the contrary, if
it has been so contaminated, as previously stated, sealing it with
collodion gives the most favorable condition for pus germs to
multiply, and so, for inflammation. Collodion is not surgically
dirty, however, like plaster, and the ether which it contains has
some antiseptic properties, so it is not really as dangerous as
plaster. A good rule to adopt is to use it only on slight, cleanly
cut wounds made by sharp instruments, and to have it removed by
a surgeon if inflammation occurs. A very good wound dressing
may be made with a few layers of antiseptic gauze placed over the
wound and attached to the skin by collodion at the edges, no collodion being put over the wound itself.

SPLINTS.

Splints are used to prevent movement at the point where a bone is broken. They must, therefore, be made of a stiff and rigid material. For first-aid purposes splints must generally be improvised from something which may easily be procured on the spot. Such articles are pieces of wood, broom handles, laths, rules, squares, wire netting, heavy cardboard, umbrellas, canes, pick handles, spades, rolls made of blankets or cloth, pillows alone or with pieces of board outside, rifles, swords and bayonets. With a broken leg it is even possible to use the other leg as a splint.

In improvising splints a few precautions should be observed. Besides being rigid enough to prevent movement at the point where a bone is broken, they should be long enough to prevent movement at the nearest joints, as this will move the broken bone and they should be as wide as the limb to which they are applied, as otherwise the bandages holding them on will press on the limb as well as on the splint and thus cause pain and perhaps displace the ends of the broken bone. On account of the danger from swelling and in order to promote the comfort of the patient and not to rub the skin, splints should be well padded on the inner side with some soft material. The clothing sometimes answers this purpose fairly well when it is not removed. Substances generally used are cotton batting, waste, tow, flannel, pieces of cloth, grass, etc. If splints are not well padded, the limb to which they are applied must be watched with special care because the swelling is likely to make the splints too tight which will cut off the circulation and may cause mortification.

TOURNIQUETS.

Tourniquets are instruments used to stop bleeding from an artery. Each has a strap to go around the limb, a pad to place on the artery and some means by which the pad may be made to press on the artery and thus stop the flow of blood. In an improvised tourniquet, which is the type most commonly used, the strap may be made of a handkerchief, towel, bandage or cravat, and a smooth round stone, a cork or some object of similar shape and size may be used for the pad. The stone, etc., had best be wrapped in a small piece of cloth so that it will not bruise the skin too much. It is then placed over the artery above the wound and the strap is best passed twice around the limb and tied loosely at its outer side. A stick is introduced between the two layers thus formed and is twisted around until the bleeding is stopped. If desired, another bandage may be used to loop over and to hold the end of the stick from twisting back and so relieving the pressure of the pad on the artery. One layer of bandage may be used for the strap if more is not procurable. In order to avoid bruising in using this it is best after introducing the stick into the loop to twist away from the body. This is illustrated under the heading Hemorrhage.

Besides the bruising of the muscles and skin which is certain to occur to some extent with any tourniquet, there is a much graver danger connected with their use. This is due to the fact that in consequence of cutting off the circulation, mortification and death of the part may follow. If a tourniquet has been in place for an hour, therefore, it is desirable to loosen it and to allow it to remain loose if no bleeding occurs. It should not be removed as it may be necessary to tighten it again quickly should bleeding recommence. Whenever a tourniquet is used, a doctor should be sent for as quickly as possible, for if 3 or 4 hours pass with a tourniquet in place, mortification is very liable to follow.

Instead of tourniquets, appliances to make pressure on the whole circumference of a limb and thus to stop bleeding are sometimes employed. The strap which has just been described, without the pad, may be used for this purpose. A special elastic bandage and elastic suspenders have also been recommended. When possible, however, use the tourniquet, as cutting off the whole circulation by pressure on the entire circumference of a limb is much more likely to cause mortification than the tourniquet, which presses to the greatest extent on the artery alone. If circular constriction is used it should not be employed for over an hour.

HEAT.

Heat employed externally is such a very valuable stimulant that every first-aid student should know how to make use of it. The ordinary hot-water bag is most convenient for this purpose, but glass bottles and jars are good. They should be covered with cloth or paper to prevent them from burning the patient. Hot bricks and stones are also useful. In using heat in this way it must be remembered that, especially with an unconscious person, there is considerable danger of causing severe burns, so one must make sure by testing the bottle, etc., on his arm or face, that it will not burn even if left in contact with the skin for some time. In applying heat by means of the objects mentioned, to get the greatest effect, they should be placed between the legs, at their outer sides and between the body and the arms. A light hot water bag lying over the heart acts as a special stimulant to it. The full hot bath— not warm, but actually hot—while effective as a stimulant, is more difficult to use than the hot-water bottles, etc., though it is well to remember that it may be employed for this purpose.

Heat applied locally causes the blood-vessels to enlarge momentarily and then to contract. Every one knows how shrunken the hands look after they have been in hot water for some time. For this reason heat may be used in congestion, too much blood in a part, or in inflammation. Cloths wrung out in very hot water are usually employed for this purpose.

COLD.

Cold as well as heat is used in first-aid work. It is employed for three important purposes: first, to reduce the temperature of the

4

body; second, to contract the blood-vessels locally and, third, to stimulate the respiration or breathing.

While the full cold or ice bath is the best method of applying cold to reduce the temperature, cold may also be used for this purpose by placing bags filled with ice around the body. Sheets wrung out in cold or ice-water wrapped around the patient, may also be used. They should never be covered with a blanket, for in this case they will soon become heated from the heat of the body and instead of a cold bath a hot steam or Russian bath will result. In using cold to reduce the temperature it should be remembered that it drives the blood from the surface of the body to the internal organs and so causes shock, and that for this reason the body must be constantly rubbed to bring the blood back to the surface.

Cold may be applied locally in any case of congestion or inflammation to contract the blood-vessels; swelling after an injury is limited by this same action of cold. It always seems strange that the two opposites—cold and heat—should have the same effect on the blood-vessels, but this is actually the case. Cold is generally preferred to heat for this purpose, however, at least in all recent cases, such as those which are cared for by first-aid students. Ice bags, cold water running from a tap, cold water in a basin or pail or cloths wrung out in cold water are generally used for this purpose. Cold metal, such as a wide knife-blade, sometimes proves a convenient means of applying cold.

Everybody knows that on jumping into cold water or on being struck by a stream of cold water he involuntarily takes a deep breath. This is due to the fact that the cold acts on the nerves of the skin and they convey the impulse to the brain, which transfers it to the respiratory organs. This so-called reflex action produced by cold is taken advantage of to cause breathing to start when it has stopped or to quicken and deepen it if it is slow and shallow. For this purpose cold water should be sprinkled on the face—the front of the body, the chest and the abdomen are particularly sensitive. Fanning increases the effect of cold used in this way, as it hastens evaporation.

STIMULANTS.

All stimulants taken internally are best given hot when possible, as aside from the particular stimulant used, heat itself is a powerful stimulant whether employed internally or externally. Safe and easily procurable stimulants are tea and coffee, a glass of wine, a dessertspoonful of whisky or brandy with an equal quantity of water, or a teaspoonful of pure alcohol with three times the quantity of water (not wood alcohol or denatured alcohol, which are poisons). These doses are for adults; half-grown children may be given half as much, and young children not over one-sixth as much. For babies three or four drops of brandy or whisky are sufficient.

Alcohol in some form may usually be easily procured and this use of alcohol is, of course, purely a medicinal one which has nothing to do with the question of the habitual drinking of alcoholic liquors. But many people object to the use of alcohol under any circumstances, and for other reasons it is not advisable to carry whisky or brandy for first-aid purposes. Aromatic spirits of ammonia which has none of the disadvantages of alcohol fulfills this need better than any other stimulant. It is best given in 20-drop to half-teaspoonful doses in one-third of a glass of hot water.

EMETICS.

It is necessary to know a few simple and easy methods to cause vomiting.

Running the finger down the throat or drinking a large quantity of warm water are usually effective. A teaspoonful of mustard or salt in a cupful of warm water are household remedies of value and the wine or syrup of ipecac are usually easily procured. The last are given in doses of from one to two teaspoonsful.

CHAPTER IV.

GENERAL DIRECTIONS FOR RENDERING FIRST AID.

In actually giving first aid several points must be taken into account. In case of accident or sudden illness when no doctor is present the man trained in first-aid work occupies for the time being the same position as a physician. For this reason in justice to his patient and to himself he must take control of matters. In a crowd, well meaning and sympathetic, but ignorant people will almost always be found, who in their desire to help may actually do a great deal of harm if they are permitted to interfere. Some firmness will be necessary to get rid of them and of the merely curious. By the exercise of tact, aided whenever possible by the display of a first-aid certificate, there will usually be no great difficulty in getting a patient in one's own charge. The patient's recovery always depends to some extent on his having plenty of fresh air, so persons should be told this and requested to clear a space around him. The only persons who should be near a patient are those actually needed to help him. If an accident occurs on the street it will sometimes be found better to take the patient to a nearby building. Do not be hurried into doing so, however, and always make sure, first, that the patient is not going to be injured by being moved. Broken bones must always be secured before a patient is moved.

If the services of a doctor are procurable, it is best to send for one at once. Sometimes it will be possible to inform the messenger of the character of the illness or injury in order that he may tell the

doctor and the latter may come prepared to treat the particular
. case, but only under exceptional conditions is it suitable to delay
the messenger for this purpose. The doctor may generally be de-
pended on to take the necessary measures on his arrival which
should not be delayed to send information which may or may not
prove of value. What has just been said of course assumes that
a physician will be sent for in all emergency cases of illness and injury. This certainly should be the rule followed whenever the
services of a physician are procurable and the accident is of sufficient moment to justify calling one. Moreover, if any doubt exists
in regard to the latter point, it is best to send for a physician. In
this connection it should be remembered that injuries and emergencies which are apparently trivial may sometimes, if not treated
promptly by a doctor, have serious consequences, and that a physician called in time may with comparative ease prevent conditions which when fully established are beyond the help of medical
science.

In approaching the patient do so calmly and without hurry.
Be quiet and cool. Unnecessary motions and loud talk impress
no one and are absolutely out of place. Generally speaking, the
first thing to do for the patient is to get him into a safe and comfortable position. The best position, unless there is some reason
to the contrary, is on the back with the head low. Never raise the
head more than necessary to put a small pillow, such as one made
of a folded coat, under it. With a flushed face, the head may be
raised to this extent; with a pale face, it should not be raised at all.
If a person is vomiting, he should be placed on his side or his head
should be turned to one side, so that the matter vomited will not
go into his wind-pipe and choke him. It should also be remembered
that unconscious persons cannot swallow and so they should never
be given water, stimulants, etc., as these will choke them by entering the wind-pipe. Slight cases of illness and injury may sit up,

but one must be sure that all serious cases are kept in the lying position.

Tight clothing interferes with both breathing and circulation. The collar should be loosened at once and when required no sense of false modesty should prevent loosening the belt and suspenders, or the waist band and the corsets.

A sick or hurt person will frequently ask for water, which may be given him with perfect safety. Cold water is usually more refreshing, but whether cold or hot, it must be given fairly slowly so that the patient has time to swallow between sips. Stimulants have already been discussed. To neglect giving a stimulant when it is required would be a grave error of judgment. The first thought with many people, however, is to procure whisky or brandy for every sufferer from illness or injury. These are really as unnecessary for every case as would be the application of splints to the leg of every injured man. They should never be given in injuries of the head, and it should be remembered that while a small quantity of liquor acts as a stimulant, that large ones are depressing.

Whatever the injury may be, it must be seen clearly before any attempt is made to treat it. In order to do this it will generally be necessary to remove some of the clothing. This is likely to be a very painful and possibly a dangerous process for the patient unless he is handled with the greatest gentleness. In removing clothing, rip up the nearest seam in the outer clothing and cut or tear the underclothing. The sound side should be undressed first, so that the injured side will be subjected to less movement. In injuries to the foot and ankle it will rarely be possible to remove the boots or shoes without giving severe pain and perhaps doing considerable damage, so they should be cut freely when this is necessary.

CHAPTER V.

SHOCK.

Description.

Shock is a more or less profound depression of the nervous system. It is sometimes called collapse.

Causes.

Usually a severe injury. Some persons are sensitive to shock, however, and so with them more shock will follow a slight injury than is the case with a severe injury in less sensitive persons.

Prevention.

The prevention of accidents, especially severe accidents. Also do not allow an injured person to see his own injury, as this is apt to increase shock. This is especially true with severe bleeding.

Symptoms.

Usually appear immediately after an injury.
Patient is more or less stupid and takes no interest in what is happening near him.
May be partly or totally unconscious or mind may wander.
Face is pale, anxious and pinched; eye-lids droop; eyes are dull, with dilated pupils.
Skin is cold.
Breathing is feeble and shallow.
Pulse is rapid and feeble and may not be able to feel at the wrist.
Usually patient gradually improves, in a few hours be-

55

coming more like himself, but may not do so, but die of heart failure.

Treatment.

Send for doctor immediately if possible. Combat depression and warm and stimulate in every possible way before arrival of doctor.

First, place patient on back with head low so that plenty of blood will enter brain.

Stimulants should always be given if patient is able to swallow. Hot coffee, hot tea or half a teaspoonful of aromatic spirits of ammonia in a tablespoonful of water. Whisky may be only stimulant procurable. If used, give one large drink only, as more is likely to cause depression.

Ammonia or smelling salts to nose.

Never remove more clothing than necessary from an injured person as this will cause more severe shock, and when possible spread coats or blankets over him.

Place hot-water bottles or hot bricks around patient when possible; flannels wrung out in hot water applied to abdomen and chest have the same effect.

Rubbing legs and arms toward body, under blankets, quickens circulation and is useful. Be careful while doing this not to uncover patient.

Warning.

While shock is so extremely common in injuries that it should always be kept in mind and treated, it must not be forgotten that something more dangerous even than shock may require attention. The symptoms of severe bleeding are very like shock, and if shock only is treated in such a case and the bleeding is not stopped the patient may very readily bleed to death.

CHAPTER VI.

COMMON ACCIDENTS AND INJURIES.

1. BRUISES, STRAINS, SPRAINS, DISLOCATIONS AND FRACTURES.
2. WOUNDS, INCLUDING TETANUS OR LOCK-JAW AND RABIES
OR THE BITES OF MAD DOGS, AND HEMORRHAGE. 3. IN-
JURIES OF AND FOREIGN BODIES IN THE EYE, EAR, NOSE AND
THROAT. 4. BURNS AND SCALDS. 5. UNCONSCIOUSNESS FROM
VARIOUS CAUSES. 6. FITS OR CONVULSIONS. 7. POISONING.
8. SUN STROKE AND HEAT EXHAUSTION. 9. FROST BITE
AND FREEZING. 10. ELECTRICITY AND LIGHTNING STROKE.
EMERGENCY SUPPLIES.

1. BRUISES, STRAINS, SPRAINS, DISLOCATIONS AND FRACTURES.

Causes.

These injuries are all caused by external violence in the form of blows or falls or by wrenching the body.

This does not apply to all compound fractures, however, as will be seen later.

Prevention.

Every one is liable to these, the commonest of injuries, and they occur under so many different circumstances that it is impossible to suggest other than the most general means for preventing them. It is safe to say, however, that a great many of them result from carelessness and that especially in dangerous places, such as the crowded streets of a city, people should be more alive to their surroundings. In other words, they should always exercise common care.

Many usual practices, such as jumping on and off trolley cars in motion, frequently cause such injuries, and the more general observance of posted directions in all situations will well repay the public. Such directions are not arbitrary, as they are, unfortunately, sometimes regarded, but represent the teachings of experience.

BRUISES.

Description.

These are perhaps the most common injuries. When a person falls and strikes some part of his body or when he is struck by something usually the skin is not broken but the force of the blow or fall injures the tissues immediately beneath the skin breaking numbers of small blood-vessels therein. Blood escapes from these small vessels and this causes the swelling and the ordinary black-and-blue spot which is due to the blood which has escaped.

Causes.

Blows or falls.

Prevention.

As given above under general heading.

Symptoms.

Pain at once from injury to nerves.

Swelling from escape of blood from vessels.

Black-and-blue spot from same cause.

Pain also later from pressure of this blood on sensitive nerves.

Pain increased by movement.

Treatment.

Slight, no treatment.

More severe, object is to limit swelling and to decrease pain.

At once: Ice or very hot or very cold water, or half alcohol and half water. Arnica or witch-hazel. These contract blood-vessels and so prevent escape of more blood and also deaden nerves to some extent, thus relieving pain. Ice may be applied directly to injured part. Best in using liquid remedy to wet cloth with liquid and then to apply cloth.

Raising bruised part diminishes pain, as it diminishes the blood-supply to the part.

In arm, when severe and movement is painful, use a sling.

No doctor is usually required for a bruise.

Warning.

A bruise may be only the least important part of an injury. So with a bruise always try to make sure there is no other injury, such as a fracture.

Bruises of the chest and abdomen sometimes result in internal injuries. They may be very dangerous from breaking of the blood-vessels of the lungs, of the abdominal organs, or from actual rupture of the soft internal structures. Severe bruises of this character therefore demand the immediate attention of a physician. In case shock is very severe after a bruise of the abdomen or chest, serious injury of the internal organs may be suspected.

STRAINS.

Description.

A strain is the name given to the injury produced by overstretching of a muscle. In severe strains small blood-vessels in the muscles are often broken so that blood escapes into the muscles in the same way that with a bruise blood escapes beneath the skin. The commonest strains are of the muscles of the back and shoulders and of the small tendons of the wrist and ankle.

Cause.

Usually a sudden wrench—may be due to lifting too heavy a weight.

Prevention.

As given above.

Symptoms.

Pain increased on movement.

Stiffness.

Lameness.

More or less swelling.

Treatment.

Not necessary to call doctor unless severe.

Absolute rest at first.

Alcohol and water, arnica and witch-hazel gently rubbed in to deaden pain. Rubbing should always be toward body. Later such rubbing may be harder to help absorption and to make strained muscles more supple.

When pain and stiffness have improved, gentle movement until both have entirely disappeared.

SPRAINS.

Description.

Sprains are injuries of joints. They result from violent stretching, twisting and partial breaking of the ligaments about a joint and are sometimes accompanied by actual breaking of the bones. The twisting or stretching results in breaking of the blood-vessels and the escape of blood and of blood-serum (the liquid part of the blood) both around and in the joint.

Sprains of the wrist and ankle are most common.

Cause.

Unnatural movement of a joint. Sometimes the cause is apparently a slight one, such as twisting the foot in stepping from the curb to the street.

Prevention.

See above under general heading.

Symptoms.

Severe pain immediately.

Pain is much increased by movement of the joint.

Swelling of joint.

Bones are not out of place and there is no deformity other than that due to swelling.

Shock, when severe.

Treatment.

Call doctor always when severe or when in doubt.

Always begin treatment at once whether doctor has been called or not.

Absolute rest in order not to do more damage by rubbing of the injured joint surfaces. This means that the patient should not be allowed to move the joint or to step on it.

Elevate joint when possible and apply heat or cold. Less blood will come to the injured joint if it is elevated and heat or cold contracts the vessels and thus limits the escape of blood and serum. Cold may be applied in the form of snow or crushed ice in a cloth. It is usually better to use cloths wrung out in very hot or very cold water or to shower the joint with very hot or cold water.

Putting sprained joint under a cold or hot water tap is also excellent.

Either heat or cold should be made use of sufficiently long to get full benefit from it, that is to say, from 24 to 48 hours. At first on the application of either heat or cold, the pain may increase, but after an hour, at the latest, it will commence to improve and will finally disappear.

Remember there may be shock and, if so, treat.

Warning.

A severe sprain, especially a sprain of the ankle, is by no means a trivial injury but one which demands the services of a physician.

DISLOCATIONS.

Description.

Dislocations are injuries of joints and are due to the head of a bone slipping out of its socket. A dislocation cannot occur, except in a joint which has been dislocated before, without tearing the ligaments which keep the joint close. Some persons, however, on account of frequent dislocations of the same joint have its ligaments so stretched that not only is dislocation easy, but no further injury of the ligaments results from it. By far the most frequent dislocation is that of the shoulder-joint, which occurs in one-half of all cases of dislocation. But dislocations of the hip-joint, the jaw and the fingers are not particularly uncommon.

Causes.

Dislocations are usually caused by a blow or a fall, but sometimes result from a violent muscular effect, such as throwing a ball.

Prevention.

As given under general heading.

Symptoms.

Deformity; that is, the joint has an unusual appearance, because the head of the bone is not in its proper place. This may be best recognized by comparing the injured with the uninjured side of the body.

The limb in which a joint is dislocated may be either longer or shorter than the uninjured limb. This depends on the direction in which the dislocation has taken place. The head of a dislocated bone may often be felt out of its place.

Limited movement as the displaced head of the bone is tightly held in its new position.

Pain from pressure of the displaced head of the bone on sensitive nerves.

Swelling from bruising of the soft parts by the displaced head of the bone.

Shock.

Treatment.

Send for a doctor at once.

Await his arrival except in dislocations of the jaw, the fingers and the shoulder without attempting to reduce dislocation.

Remember that attempts to reduce dislocations, other than those of the fingers and the jaw, by one not familiar with anatomy may result in great harm to the patient, for the movements necessary to do so may cause serious injury to the blood-vessels, nerves and soft parts.

When no attempt is made to reduce the dislocation, the patient should be put in a comfortable position and the injured joint should be covered with cloths wrung out in

very hot or very cold water so as to contract the vessels
and to prevent swelling as much as possible.

Dislocation of the Lower Jaw.

This may usually be successfully treated by almost any
one. This is fortunate, as a dislocated jaw with the
open mouth in consequence is most painful and uncomfortable   To reduce a dislocation of the jaw, both
thumbs must first be wrapped in several layers of cloth
so that they will not be liable to injury. Both thumbs
are then placed in the patient's mouth resting on his
lower teeth on each side while the fingers seize the
lower jaw outside. First pressure is made downward
and then backward. As soon as the jaw starts into
place the thumbs should be slid off the teeth to the inside
of the cheeks or they will be caught between the teeth
when the jaw springs into place. The overstretched
muscles act just like a rubber band and one must be
quick or his thumbs will be injured. When dislocation
is reduced put on jaw bandage.

Dislocation of the Fingers.

These, not including those of the second joint of the
thumb, present no great difficulties to the first-aid student.
The dislocated finger should first be grasped firmly on
the hand side. The end of the finger should then be
pulled straight out away from the hand and the bone
will usually slip into place. No bandage will be required.

Dislocation of the Shoulder.

No attempt should be made to reduce this dislocation
if the services of a physician can be obtained within a

reasonable time, say four hours. Make your decision on this point at once, for if you are compelled by circumstances to attempt to reduce the dislocation you must get to work immediately before the muscles have become set and rigid from the irritation caused by the displaced head of the bone.

Frequently little difficulty will be experienced in reducing a dislocation of the shoulder, especially if the joint has been dislocated before. To accomplish it, the patient should be made to lie down flat on his back. The person who is going to try to reduce the dislocation should then sit down beside him on the injured side facing toward his head and should place his inner heel, after the shoe has been removed, in the arm-pit of the patient's injured side and then draw down the dislocated arm and drag it toward the uninjured side at the same time pressing outward and upward with the heel. This will usually pry the end of the dislocated bone outward, and as soon as it is free it will snap back into place. In order to keep the bone in place, the arm should then be bandaged to the side with the forearm carried across the chest and the hand placed on the opposite shoulder.

Warning.

In case much difficulty is experienced in reducing any dislocation, do not persist in trying to do so.

FRACTURES.

Description.

When a bone is broken, the injury is called a fracture. Our bones are brittle and when the force used against them is sufficient they break much as would a dry stick. Fractures are among the commonest injuries, ten times

5

as common as dislocations. About two thirds of all fractures are of the bones of the limbs. Next in frequency are those of the collar-bone and ribs. Fractures of the skull, spine and pelvis are comparatively rare.

A simple fracture is one in which the skin is not pierced.

A compound fracture is one in which the skin is pierced.

Causes.

Simple: blows and falls. Compound: also,—from bad handling of simple fractures and from wounds.

Prevention.

Simple: as given under general heading. Compound: also,—by proper handling of simple fractures and the prevention of wounds.

Symptoms.   Simple Fracture.

History of blow or fall.

Pain at point of fracture.

Tenderness at point of fracture.

Person injured is unable to move fractured limb.

Deformity. With a fracture a limb will be altered in shape and shortened or bent. Always compare with the uninjured side.

Recognition by touch, an inequality may often be felt by running finger along a broken bone.

Loss of rigidity of bone. On moving a limb in which bone is fractured, instead of the bone being moved as a whole it will be noticed that at the point of fracture there is unusual movement, something like that of a hinge.

Crepitas. This is the surgical term applied to the grating which is heard or felt when the broken ends of the bone are rubbed on each other.

Shock.

Warning.

As one may do great harm by moving a broken bone, for the broken ends are likely to be very sharp, it is much safer when an injured person is unable to move a limb, and from appearances it seems probable that a fracture has occurred, to conclude that it is a fracture without further examination, and to so treat it.

Treatment. Simple Fracture.

Send for a doctor.

The object of treatment before his arrival is to prevent further injury, especially puncture of the skin by the sharp, knife-like edges of the broken bone. If this occurs the simple fracture is, of course, converted into a compound fracture. In the former injury there is no chance of wound infection as the unbroken skin prevents germs from reaching the break in the bone, while in the latter the skin is cut through and in consequence germs reach the broken bone ends and infection occurs. So instead of the few weeks of comparatively painless healing of the simple fracture without much danger, a compound fracture is caused with probable wound infection, inflammation, pus or matter, and perhaps months of sickness from blood-poisoning, with considerable danger of death. In the treatment of simple fractures the primary object is accomplished by preventing movement of the ends of the broken bone.

If the doctor may be expected to arrive promptly, nothing need be done except to put the patient in a comfortable position. If it is evident that in order to do this the broken bone will be moved, it must be supported firmly by the hands. One hand should support the broken bone on each side of the break. The bone must not bend at the break while the patient changes his position to a more comfortable one. Then the broken bone had best be supported in the natural position on a pillow or a folded coat. In so supporting it great care must be taken that it is not bent or does not drag on the point of fracture.

If the patient must be moved more than slightly, as just described, the broken bone should be set; that is to say, it should be gently drawn into its natural position, always determining this by comparing it with the opposite side, and held there firmly by the application of splints.

If the injured person is wearing thin summer clothing, it will not usually be necessary to remove the clothing in order to examine for fracture. In fact, it will be better not to try to do so, as this may result in injury from moving the sharp ends of the bone, and when the clothing is left on it furnishes excellent padding for splints. With thick clothing, however, very likely one will not be able to tell that a fracture has occurred or what the character of the injury is. In this case never try to take off the clothing, but cut it in the seams with a sharp knife or scissors.

Treat shock.

Symptoms. Compound Fracture.

Besides the symptoms already described, there is a wound leading down to the broken bone, or the broken end of the bone protrudes through the skin.

Treatment. Compound Fracture.

Send for doctor.

Expose fracture by cutting clothing.

Turn back clothing from wound.

Use same precaution as in simple fracture to prevent movement of sharp ends of broken bone.

Do not touch wound with fingers or anything else.

As soon as possible procure an antiseptic or surgically clean compress and place it on the wound.

If sharp bone is buttoned-holed through the skin, as frequently happens, do not attempt to restore it to its

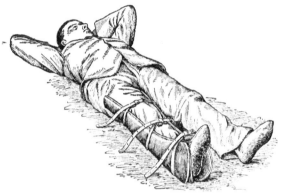

FIG. 23.—Splint for fracture of lower leg. (*Drill Regulations, H. C., U. S. A.*)

place, but by padding splint hold it in position as it is.

Always treat wound first, then fracture.

Treat shock.

Warning.

Never in any fracture attempt to transport patient until broken bone is firmly fixed in position by splints.

Fracture of Lower Leg.

Symptoms.

As given above.   Patient falls to ground.   Is not usually difficult to detect fracture.

Treatment.

Send for doctor.

Secure pillow, sack stuffed like pillow with hay, straw or the like or a blanket rolled on poles at each side so as to make trough.

Gently lift leg to pillow, etc., placing one hand above and the other below break under leg, always holding in natural position.

Leg on pillow, should not allow toe to turn in or out, but should be supported in same position as toe of uninjured leg.

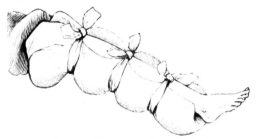

Fig. 24.—The pillow splint. (*Dulles.*)

Nothing further unless must move patient. If this must be done the leg should be drawn into natural position and splinted. Use two splints when procurable. Though any stiff material may be used for these splints, preferably they should be of thin boards longer than the leg so as to prevent movement at the knee-joint, and wider than leg is thick. The splints should be applied outside of pillow, one at the inner and the other at outer side of leg. They should be held in place by 3 or 4 strips of cloth, straps or handkerchiefs passed around splints, pillow and leg and tied.   Care must be taken that none of these strips are directly over break, as this will cause intense pain by pressure.   The pillow alone makes a fairly good support even without splints.   Splints also may be used without a pillow.   If this is done the clothing, straw, hay, cotton, leaves or something else soft must be used for padding under the splints, which are tied in place in the way described above.

In case of emergency anything stiff of sufficient length, such as a cane, umbrella or the like, may be used for the outer splint, the other leg being used for the inner splint.   The strips of cloth or handkerchiefs are then passed around the splint and both legs and tied as before.

Treat Shock.

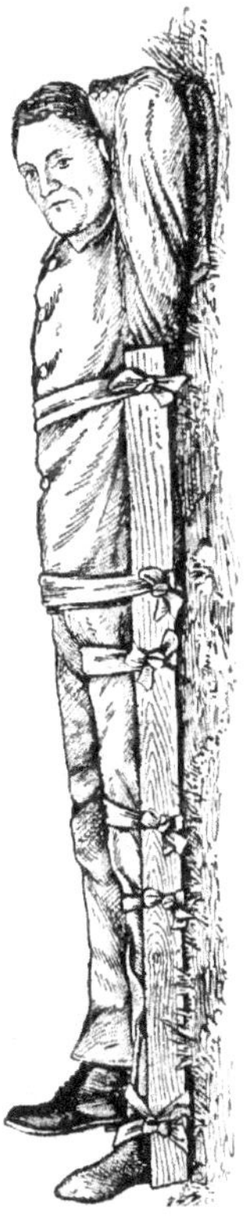

Fracture of Thigh.

Symptoms.

As above, patient falls to ground. May be difficult to detect fracture on account of thick muscles.

Treatment.

The necessity of procuring a physician and of treating shock are greater than in fracture of the leg.   Remarks in reference to careful handling of broken bone apply. If difficult to detect fracture, treat as fracture.

FIG. 25.—Splint for fracture of thigh. (*Drill Regulations, H. C., U. S. A.*)

A long splint extending in a solid piece from foot to arm-pit is required for outside splint to prevent movement of thigh-joint. This should be firmly fixed by encircling strips of cloth to the chest as well as to the limb.

Inner splint had best extend from crotch to foot. If no inner splint can be obtained, tie legs and thighs together.

Broken Knee-cap.

Symptoms.

As above, patient falls to ground and cannot raise leg. Not difficult to detect fracture, as can feel groove in knee-cap immediately beneath the skin.

Treatment.

Services of a physician will be required and shock generally demands treatment. Must also use care in moving leg.

Straighten leg.

Secure splint long enough to extend from middle of thigh to middle of lower leg. Preferably, this should be a thin board as wide as thigh, but a cane, umbrella or the like may be used in case of emergency. Make pad for splint, apply splint to back of thigh and leg with middle opposite bend of knee and tie in place with strips of cloth or handkerchiefs. Be careful not to put bandage over break, but one strip immediately above and one immediately below knee.

Fracture of Collar-bone.

Symptoms.

Patient supports elbow of injured side with hand of other side.

Is unable to raise arm above shoulder.

Is easy to feel depression by running finger over injured collar-bone.

Treatment.

Send for doctor.

Make pad from a large handkerchief, two medium-sized handkerchiefs, a triangular bandage or the like.

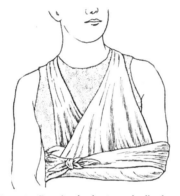

FIG. 26.—Dressing for fracture of collar-bone.

Place this pad in arm-pit of injured side. Put arm in sling with forearm at right angle to upper arm.

Take a bandage about 3 inches wide, put this horizontally around body and injured arm at elbow. It will, of course, encircle both the elbow, the bent arm and the body. When tied by pulling elbow to body it will force upper end of humerus outward.

Another method:

Have patient lie down and place his injured shoulder on pillow in a comfortable position till doctor arrives.

Treat shock.

Fracture of Upper Arm and Forearm.

Symptoms.

These fractures can almost always be easily detected by the symptoms already given.

Treatment.

Send for doctor.

Treat shock.

Gently straighten limb so as to put it in natural position.

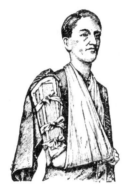

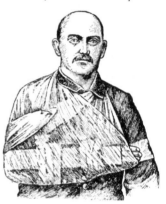

Fig. 27.—Fracture of upper arm. (*Drill Regulations, H. C., U. S. A.*)

Fig. 28.—Splint and sling for forearm. (*Drill Regulations, H. C., U. S. A.*)

Secure two splints long enough, in upper arm to extend from shoulder and arm-pit to elbow, and in forearm from elbow to middle of hand. These are best flat boards, shingles are excellent, but may be of any stiff material, such as twigs, cover of wine bottles, tin trough, etc.

Pad splints well.

In upper arm, if lower part of bone is broken, apply one

splint behind and the other in front. If fracture is of middle or upper part, apply one splint to inner and the other to outer side of arm.

Support by sling.

In forearm:

Place forearm across the chest, thumb up.

Apply one padded splint—clothing will do for padding—to outer side from elbow to beyond wrist and the other to inner surface extending to tips of fingers.

Support by sling.

Broken Wrist.

This is an extremely common injury resulting from falls on the hands which are put out in falling forward to protect the body.

Symptoms.

This belongs to a class of fractures to which the name impacted is given. The force of the injury actually drives one bone into the other so that they are held together.

Great deformity, no crepitas, movement, etc.

Treatment.

Send for doctor.

Do not attempt to free bones, but leave them as they are. Otherwise treat like fracture of forearm.

Broken Fingers.

Symptoms.

Usual symptoms of fracture, which is easily detected.

Treatment.

Gently draw into natural position.

Put narrow padded splint under finger and hold it in place with a narrow bandage.

Support hand in sling.

Show to doctor as early as practicable.

Fracture of Ribs.

Symptoms.

Sharp pain on taking a long breath or coughing. Breathing is usually short, patient often presses hand to side to prevent movement of chest.

May feel grating of ends of broken bones on each other by placing hand on chest at point where pain is most severe.

Treatment.

Tie a large handkerchief or a triangular bandage firmly around the chest, pin a large towel snugly around chest or apply a roller bandage to chest. These limit chest motion and thus diminish pain.

If shock is severe, call doctor immediately. If not, after bandage is in place may visit a doctor as soon as practicable. Treat shock.

Fracture of Skull.

Symptoms.

Patient probably unconscious from injury to brain. If at base of skull, there will probably be a discharge of blood from nose, ears or mouth. If at vault, fracture can easily be detected under skin.

Treatment.

Send for doctor.

Place in lying-down position with head slightly raised and keep very quiet until doctor arrives.

Fracture of Lower Jaw.

Symptoms.

Mouth open, patient cannot speak.

Fracture may often be felt outside, and inside there will be an irregularity of the teeth.

May be bleeding from gums.

Shock.

Treatment.

Send for doctor.

Gently raise broken jaw and bring lower against upper teeth.

Support in this position with the jaw bandage described on page 39 or with two strips of bandage, one vertical, tied over top of head and the other longer, brought to back of head, crossed and brought horizontally to forehead and tied there.

Treat shock.

Fracture of Nose.

Symptoms.

Usually not difficult to detect.

Pain, swelling, crepitas and deformity. Swelling may be so great that obscures deformity.

Is not infrequently compound.

Treatment.

Put in as natural position as possible and hold there with an adhesive-plaster strip across nose from cheek to cheek.

Before applying plaster, put a small compress of gauze on each side of nose.

Consult doctor, as there is danger of permanent deformity.

Broken Back.

Symptoms.

Patient unable to move.

No motion or feeling of body below injury.

Treatment.

Send for doctor at once. If possible, do not move patient before his arrival.

If patient must be taken from the spot where his injury has occurred, procure ample assistance to lift him. This should be done with the greatest care so as not to bend spine for this will crush spinal cord.

Put litter under patient and gently lower him to litter.

2. WOUNDS, INCLUDING TETANUS OR LOCK-JAW AND RABIES OR THE BITES OF MAD DOGS, AND HEMORRHAGE.

Description of Wounds.

A wound is an injury in which the skin is broken and there is usually more or less damage to the tissues beneath it. This serves to distinguish wounds from the injuries which have just been described (except compound fractures, which are really wounds) for with the former the injury is confined to the tissues underneath the skin. In wounds, as the protective covering, the skin, is broken through, there is danger of the entrance of pus germs and consequently of inflammation with the formation of matter or pus. In wounds, too, as blood-vessels must be injured, there is more or less hemorrhage or bleeding.

Varieties of Wounds.

1. Cut or incised wounds, in which the skin and underlying tissues are cleanly divided by a sharp instrument. They are caused by razors, sharp knives, glass and the like. To prevent them as with the former class of injuries common care should be exercised. Carelessness on the part of men or women in handling knives or cutting instruments is bad enough, but the limit of carelessness is almost reached in allowing children to have such things. In this

variety of wounds, as blood-vessels are cleanly cut across, there is likely to be severe bleeding.

2. Torn or lacerated wounds, in which the tissues are torn rather than cut. They are caused by a tearing or crushing injury such as the blow of a blunt instrument or by being run over or struck by a wagon, trolley or railway car. As a means of prevention, attention need be called only to common care. With them, as the blood-vessels are crushed as well as the other tissues, hemorrhage is not nearly so likely to occur as in the preceding variety, but on account of the character of the injury, dirt is likely to be ground into the tissues and they are so extensively torn and destroyed that infection followed by inflammation and matter or pus is extremely common.

3. Punctured wounds are deep wounds of small calibre produced by sharp-pointed instruments, such as daggers, bayonets and the like. Wounds caused by bullets are also included in this class. Wounds of this variety are, of course, frequently purposely inflicted, but the great majority of bullet wounds in civil life results from carelessness which is almost, if not quite, criminal. "I didn't know it was loaded" is not sufficient excuse for shooting a fellow-being, and if one observes the rule of never pointing a gun or pistol at himself or at any one else he will have no occasion to make this excuse. The amount of bleeding in this variety of wounds is often slight, but may be great if a large blood-vessel is injured. Infection is not uncommon, as pus organisms when carried into such wounds have ideal conditions for multiplication.

Symptoms of Wounds.

Presence of the wound.
Pain.
Shock.
Hemorrhage.

HEMORRHAGE: Practically all wounds bleed more or less, but comparatively few are accompanied by dangerous hemorrhage, as large blood-vessels usually escape injury. Besides the actual appearance of blood in hemorrhage, the loss of a considerable amount of blood gives rise to certain symptoms: Faintness, with cold skin, pale face, dilated pupils, feeble, irregular breathing, sighing, weak pulse, dizziness and loss of consciousness. The severity of the symptoms depend on how much and how rapidly blood is lost.

Treatment of Wounds.

This had best be considered under two headings:

1. Treatment of wounds without severe hemorrhage, and
2. Treatment of wounds with severe hemorrhage.

1. Treatment of wounds without severe hemorrhage.

In deep wounds or those which cover a considerable surface, always send for a doctor at once. It is always better to call in a physician if you doubt your ability or resources.

Cut or rip clothing so as to get a view of the wound.

Turn back the clothing so it does not touch wound.

Do not touch wound yourself nor allow patient to touch it.

Remember there is no hurry, for air will not infect the wound.

If a physician may be expected to arrive within a few moments, it will usually be necessary to do nothing further. Exposure to the air is much safer than the application of anything which is not surgically clean or antiseptic. If, however, you have a surgically clean or antiseptic compress—apply it to the wound at once and bandage firmly into place. This will prevent accidental contamination and will usually stop any bleeding there may be. In fact, this procedure will stop hemorrhage in ninety-nine per cent. of all wounds.

Treat shock, if any.

If patient is faint, always have him lie down with his head low.

With trivial wounds, such as scratches, it is much better to encourage bleeding than to try to stop it.

Do not suck such wounds, but by pressure at their sides make them bleed. In the fingers this is best done by milking the finger.

Do not wipe off the blood unless you have a surgically clean cloth with which to do so. This is the only class of wounds in which water may be used to wash off the blood. The danger of contaminating these small wounds by water is very slight and the matter washed away by the water is much more dangerous than the water itself.

A piece of clean gauze makes a good dressing, or collodion may be applied.

2. **Treatment of wounds with severe hemorrhage.**

Check the bleeding.

Put patient in such a position that he will be least affected by the loss of blood. This is lying down with the head low so that the brain will get as much blood as possible. Do nothing which will increase bleeding. Violent movements must be prevented. When once the bleeding has ceased the patient should remain quiet, as any movement may dislodge the clot and start it again. Naturally, stimulants increase the force of the heart, so they are undesirable; but sometimes the patient becomes so weak that it is absolutely necessary to give them to prevent him from dying. Whenever possible, always avoid doing so

6

until the bleeding has been checked by some mechanical means.

In order to check the bleeding it is necessary to know from which kind of vessels it comes.

1. Arterial hemorrhage is recognized by bright red blood expelled in jets. The blood is lost very rapidly.

2. Venous hemorrhage is recognized by a steady flow of dark blue blood.

3. Capillary hemorrhage is characterized by the oozing of blood of a brick color.

Hemorrhage will not be severe except from arteries and large veins.

Naturally, as arteries, capillaries and veins may all be cut in a wound, there may be bleeding from all three. In this case arterial hemorrhage demands first consideration, and with venous and capillary hemorrhage the latter may be disregarded for the time being.

Arterial Hemorrhage.

Treatment.

Send for a doctor at once.

Do not wait for him, for by so doing the patient may be dead or in a hopeless condition when he arrives.

If necessary, cut off clothing at once so as to see bleeding point. In very severe hemorrhage proceed with next step before doing this.

Press with your fingers or thumb on the artery between the bleeding point and the heart. This stops the bleeding just as you can check the water flowing from a hose by pressure in any part of its length. It does more than this, however, Nature's method of checking any hemorrhage is by the formation of a clot, and as pressure prevents the washing away of the blood beyond the point of pressure an opportunity is given for a clot to form.

The points where pressure can best be made on arteries have already been given, but it will be best to review this subject so far as the principal points where pressure can be most effectively made are concerned:

The temporal artery is reached by pressure in front of the

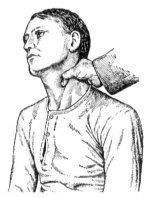 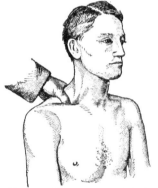

FIG. 29.—Pressure on carotid artery. (*Drill Regulations, H. C., U. S. A.*)

FIG. 30.— Pressure on subclavian artery. (*Drill Regulations, H. C., U. S. A.*)

ear just above where the lower jaw can be felt working in its socket. A branch of this artery crosses the temple on a line from the upper border of the ear to above the eye-brow. Either of these points can be used for bleeding above on the same side of the head.

The carotid artery may be compressed by pressing the thumb or fingers deeply into the neck in front of the strongly marked muscle which reaches from the upper part of the breast-bone to behind the ear. Figure 29 shows

pressure on the carotid on the left side. All bleeding
from the head, except from the side above, which has
already been referred to, had best be checked by pressure
on the carotid artery.

In bleeding from wounds of the shoulder or arm-pit, the
subclavian artery may be reached by pressing the thumb
deeply into the hollow behind the collar-bone. (Fig. 30.)

In bleeding from any part of the arm or hand, the bra-

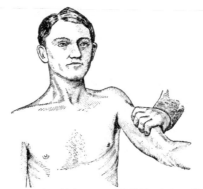

FIG. 31.—Pressure on brachial artery. (*Drill Regulations, H. C., U. S. A.*)

chial artery should be pressed outward against the bone
just behind the inner border of the large muscle of the
upper arm. (Fig. 31.)

In bleeding from the thigh, leg or foot, press backward
with the thumbs at the middle of the groin where the
artery passes over the bone. (Fig. 32.)

In making pressure in this way, if you feel the beat of the
artery, you can be quite sure that with a little care to get
it between your fingers and the hard point you can check

the bleeding. If you have stopped the bleeding in the manner just described, you may also be quite sure that the patient is safe so long as you continue the pressure. You will hardly be able to do this for more than ten or fifteen minutes, however, as your fingers will become tired and cramped. It will be best, therefore, in wounds

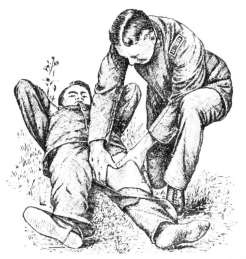

FIG. 32.—Pressure on femoral artery (correct point for pressure is higher than that illustrated.) (*Drill Regulations, H. C., U. S. A.*)

of the extremities to have a tourniquet made to place around the limb against your fingers with the pad on the artery; the tourniquet then to be twisted. Tourniquets are described on page 47. Another method which gives the same results as a tourniquet may be used in bleeding below the knee or elbow. In either a good-sized pad

made of gauze or a roll of cloth should be put in the bend
of the joint and the joint bent together and tied in this
position with a bandage or a strip of cloth so that the pad
makes pressure on the artery in the joint angle.

One of these methods will usually be all that is necessary
if the services of a doctor can be procured within two or
three hours.   If this is not the case you will be in a serious

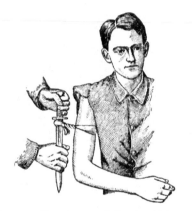

FIG. 33.—Tourniquet applied to brachial artery.
(*Drill Regulations, H.C., U. S. A.*)

position.   If either apparatus is left in place much longer
than this there is considerable danger from cutting off the
blood-supply that you will cause the death of the part
below.   No part of the body can do without blood for a
long period, and yet if the pressure is removed the bleeding   may   recommence.   Under   such   circumstances,
therefore, leave the tourniquet or pad in position as long as
you dare, say two hours.   In the meantime procure an

antiseptic compress or have one prepared in the manner already described. Place this gently on the wound and bandage firmly in place so as to make strong pressure on the bleeding point. The pressure between the heart and

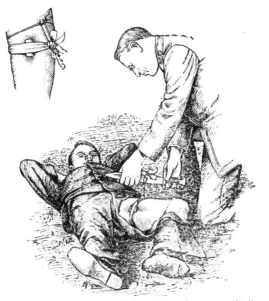

FIG. 34.—Tourniquet applied to femoral artery. (Drill Regulations, H. C., U. S. A.)

the wound may now be gradually released. If the bleed ing does not recommence, well and good; if it does, the tourniquet or pad must be reapplied. Another attempt to remove it should not be made for at least an hour, as time is needed for the clot to reform.

Suppose, at first, and this is by no means improbable, that you have failed to stop the bleeding by pressure between the heart and the bleeding point. There is still no reason why you should become panic stricken. Of course you do not want to put your fingers in the wound as this will be very likely to infect it, but in case of a severe arterial hemorrhage which you are unable to check by pressure between the heart and the bleeding point you must at once make pressure on the cut artery in the wound. If you have an antiseptic compress or a surgically clean cloth to put over your fingers, which are used to make direct pressure, so much the better, as this will prevent infection; but do not wait to obtain it. When direct pressure is made in this way it should be replaced, if possible, by a compress bandaged in place in the manner which has already been described.

With wounds of the smaller arteries if a compress is firmly bandaged in the wound at the beginning it will often be all that is required to check bleeding. Position is also of value in stopping such hemorrhage. By elevating the arm or leg the heart is made to pump against gravity and a much better chance is given for a clot to form, which will block the injured artery.

Venous Hemorrhage.

(Large Veins.)

Treatment.

Stopping bleeding of this character is rather simple as compared with checking arterial hemorrhage.

Send for a doctor.

Remove any bands, such as tight collars, belts, garters

and clothing which prevent the return flow of blood to the heart.

If a limb be wounded, elevate it so as to assist the flow of blood back to the heart.

Apply a compress directly to wound and bandage on tightly.

If no compress can be obtained which is surgically clean or antiseptic, if bleeding is very severe it will be necessary to make direct pressure in the wound with the fingers. This will, of course, be done at the risk of infecting the wound.

If possible, keep wounded part in an elevated position for some hours after bleeding has stopped.

With wounds of the neck, such as those caused in an attempt to cut the throat, some of the jugular veins are often divided. It is quite probable in such a case that death will occur before anything can be done. If not, jam the fingers on the bleeding point at once and replace them with a compress at your leisure. This compress should be bandaged tightly in place.

Varicose Veins are veins which have become very large from weakening of their walls. Only those of the legs need be considered here. They may burst from injury or without an injury, causing serious or even fatal hemorrhage if they are not given prompt attention.

Send for a doctor at once.

Put patient on his back.

Remove all bands around leg above bleeding point.

Raise leg.

Cut and rip clothing so as to get at bleeding point. Turn back clothing from wound.

Place surgically clean or antiseptic compress on bleeding point and bandage firmly in position, or when absolutely necessary use fingers first for direct pressure on the bleeding point and replace them by a clean compress. Keep patient lying down for some hours with the leg elevated.

If there has been considerable loss of blood, cover patient warmly and place hot bottles around him. Give stimulants only when absolutely necessary to prevent death, as they will increase the force of the heart and so the bleeding.

Internal Hemorrhage.

May result either from a deep wound which cuts a large blood-vessel of one of the internal organs or from the bursting of a blood vessel of the lungs or stomach.

Treatment.

Send for a doctor at once.

Put patient in a lying-down position immediately, with his head lower than his body.

Apply ice or cloths wrung out in very cold water to the point from which you think the bleeding comes. To distinguish between bleeding from the lungs and stomach, remember that from the former the blood is bright red and frothy and is coughed up, while from the latter it is dark and is vomited.

Give stimulants only when patient is becoming very weak.

Nose-bleed.

Usually this does not result from a wound, but comes on spontaneously. Slight nose-bleed does not require treatment, as no harm will result from it.

Treatment. Severe.

Place patient in a chair with his head hanging backward. Loosen collar and anything tight around the neck. Apply cold to the back of the neck by means of a key or of a cloth wrung out in cold water.

Put a roll of paper under the upper lip between it and the gum.

If bleeding does not cease, salt and water, a teaspoonful of salt or vinegar to a cupful of water, should be snuffed up the nose.

If bleeding still continues, send for a doctor to come at once. Before his arrival place a small piece of cotton or gauze in the nostril from which the blood comes and shove it in gently for about one inch. A pencil answers very well to push this plug in.

Pinching the soft part of the nose below the bone will also help to stop bleeding.

Stimulants should be used only as in the other classes of hemorrhage.

Abdominal Wounds.

All wounds should be treated on the general principles already described. A word or two is required, however, on the subject of Abdominal Wounds in which more or less of the abdominal contents escape through a large cut.

Send for a doctor at once.

Place a clean cloth over the wound and keep it constantly wet with a weak solution of salt and water, for if these delicate structures become dry they will suffer almost fatal damage from this cause alone.

Treat shock.

Wounds in Which Foreign Bodies Remain.

Treatment.

Such bodies should be gently pulled from the wound in a direction contrary to that in which they entered.

If they are of considerable size and have damaged the tissues a good deal, the wound should be shown to a doctor at the earliest opportunity.

With a splinter of wood, the commonest of such foreign bodies: Pull the splinter from the wound with a pair of pinchers or by putting a knife blade against it and holding it on the blade with the thumb-nail.

The same method may be used with a splinter under the nail. But if it is broken under the nail, scrape the nail thin over it and cut out a small V-shaped piece so as to reach it.

Small splinters in the skin may be removed by a needle. In order to avoid possible infection it will be much safer to wash the skin with hot water and soap and to pass the needle through a flame before using it.

A wound from which a foreign body has been removed should never be sealed with plaster or collodion.

Tetanus or Lock-jaw.

Description.

A few words have already been said on this disease, but quite enough to show that it is caused by a germ which is introduced into the body through a wound, just as is the pus germ. Lock-jaw is a terrible disease which comes on some time after a wound is received and has as prominent symptoms, convulsions and spasms, with usually a fatal termination.

Causes.

Usually a deep wound from a rusty nail or some similar object which enters the foot or from a torn wound of the hand through which dirt is introduced.

Prevention.

Tetanus is much more common in some places than others, and in such places it is, of course, very foolish to go about barefooted. Anywhere a wound of the character described should be promptly shown to a doctor.

Treatment.

If possible, make such wounds bleed freely by pressure. Dress them with clean gauze like other wounds, but never seal them with plaster or collodion. Show them to a doctor.

Rabies (Mad Dog).

Description.

This is so-called hydrophobia and results from the bite of a mad dog. The disease is quite as terrible a one as tetanus and like it comes on some time after the injury is received. Death is almost certain unless proper treatment is given at one of the many institutions now established for this purpose.

Cause.

The bite of a dog suffering from hydrophobia.

Prevention.

Never regard the bite of a dog lightly, however slight it may be. Do not kill the dog, but have him sent, if possible, to some one who can make the necessary examination of his body, so as to find out whether or not he has hydrophobia.

Treatment.

If bitten by a dog make the wound bleed as freely as possible so as to wash out the poison. This should be done by pressure at the edges of the wound.

Cover the wound with a clean compress, but do not seal up the poison which it may contain with collodion or plaster.

Seek immediate treatment from a doctor.

3. INJURIES OF AND FOREIGN BODIES IN THE EYE, EAR, NOSE AND THROAT.

Eye.

As previously stated, the eye-ball is fairly well protected from injury, but such injuries do occasionally occur. The symptoms are severe pain and redness of the eye, and if a wound has been inflicted it is usually easy to see the cut. Such injuries should be treated by a doctor. Therefore, in any injury of the eye-ball, cover both eyes with absorbent cotton or soft cloths soaked in cool water so as to keep the eye-lids still, and bandage them into place with bandages around the head. Be careful not to put on these bandages so tightly that they will press on the eye-balls, and in order to prevent inflammation keep them constantly wet with cool water until the services of a doctor can be procured.

Splinters in the eye should be pulled out if possible. If they cannot be removed, put a few drops of olive or castor oil in the eye. Whether removed or not, the eyes should be treated in the manner just described and a doctor should be consulted as soon as possible.

Foreign bodies in the eye are usually cinders, sand or particles of dust. They cause a great deal of discomfort and pain, and tears, which, fortunately, often wash them out.

Never rub the eye, as this will be likely to rub the foreign body into its delicate covering.

First, close the eye so that the tears will accumulate and the foreign body will frequently be washed out or into view, so that it may be easily removed. If this fails, pull the upper lid over the lower two or three times, close the nostril on the opposite side with the finger and have the patient blow his nose hard.

If the foreign body still remains in the eye, examine first under the lower, then under the upper lid. For the former, have the patient look up, press the lower lid down and if the foreign body is seen brush it off with the corner of a clean handkerchief. The upper lid is not so easy to see. Seat patient in a chair with his head bent backward. Stand behind him and place a match across the upper lid one-half inch from its edge. Turn the upper lid up and back over the match and brush off the foreign body as before. A few drops of castor oil in the eye after removing a foreign body will soothe it.

Lime in the eye may be neutralized by bathing it with a solution of vinegar, a teaspoonful to a cupful of water. Particles of lime large enough to be seen should be removed like other foreign bodies.

Ear.

The treatment of injuries of the ear should be left to a doctor. It should be remembered, however, that injuries of a serious character may be caused by attempts to clean the ear with pointed instruments, and in removing wax from the ear nothing should be used except the end of the finger over which should be placed a handkerchief or towel wet with warm water. Even in using the finger, care should be taken not to crowd in into the ear, but to be gentle.

Insects or flies in the ear cause a great deal of pain and discomfort. A little warm oil dropped into the ear, the head being inclined to the opposite side, will usually kill flies and insects and they will float out.

Do nothing further, but obtain the services of a doctor, which should also be done as promptly as possible for other foreign bodies in the ear.

Nose.

It will not be necessary to discuss injuries of the nose here.

Foreign bodies, such as shoe buttons, peas and beans, are frequently put into the nose as well as the ears by children, for whom they are dangerous playthings.

If a foreign body has lodged in the nose, close the opposite nostril with the finger and have the patient blow his nose hard, or sneezing may be caused by tickling the nose with a feather. If this does not result in the foreign body being expelled, the patient should be taken to a doctor.

Throat.

Both injuries of and foreign bodies in the throat are of special interest, not because of their local effect, but because by blocking the wind-pipe they may cause suffocation.

Internal injuries of the throat may be disregarded here.

Hanging is perhaps the commonest external cause of throat injury producing suffocation.

Treatment.

Do not wait for assistance. Grasp patient around body and lift him so as to take weight off neck.

Cut rope.

Remove rope from neck.

Tear collar and waist band so as to free chest and abdomen.

Perform artificial respiration. (See page 164.)

Send some one else for doctor at once.

Do not leave patient yourself for this purpose.

Choking caused by other external causes should be
treated on the same principles so far as loosening clothing, etc., about chest and abdomen and performing artificial respiration are concerned.

Foreign bodies in throat:

Such foreign bodies are commonly pieces of meat, coins,
buttons or other hard substances, and children are naturally the most frequent sufferers.

Symptoms.

Patient gags and coughs. Frequently patient attempts
to pull out foreign body with the fingers. If he is unsuc-
cessful and the foreign body completely blocks the throat
his face will become dark red, his breathing will become
labored and he will soon become unconscious. If the
foreign body does not completely block the air-passage
the symptoms will be of the same character, but not so
severe.

Prevention.

Babies and small children should not be allowed to put
things which may block their throats into their mouths,
as a sudden inspiration will be very likely to draw them
into the air-passages.

Treatment.

A doctor should be called, but do not await his arrival.

The patient should be turned upside down at once.

Put the finger into the back of the throat and try to hook
out the foreign body. Do this boldly, for failure may
mean the death of the patient.

After foreign body has been removed, if breathing has
ceased, perform artificial respiration.

If a person merely chokes, however, because of a foreign

7

body entering the larynx without alarming symptoms of suffocation, thumping him on the back will often dislodge the foreign body and nothing more need be done.

4. BURNS AND SCALDS.

Description.

Burns result from exposure of the body to dry heat, such as a fire, while scalds are produced by moist heat in the form of hot water, steam, etc. With either, the injury may be confined to the skin alone or it may extend deeper. With burns all the tissues of the body may be charred down to the bone and with scalds all the tissues may be actually cooked. With either the danger will depend upon the depth, extent and part injured as well as on the age of the injured person. Both burns and scalds of the throat and wind-pipe are especially dangerous, as the swelling of the injured part is likely to result in suffocation.

Cause.

Burns: Flames or fires, hot or molten metal and explosions of gas or gunpowder.

Scalds: Steam, boiling water or hot oil.

Prevention.

The prevention of burns and scalds is rather a complicated subject, as it involves: (1) Prevention of fires. (2) Putting out fires. (3) Rescue of persons at fires. (4) Extinguishing burning clothing. (5) Preventing burns and scalds from hot stoves, cooking utensils, etc. (6) Avoidance of danger from hot or molten metal; and (7) Methods to prevent explosions of gas and gunpowder.

Prevention of Fires.

Many fires result from carelessness. Never throw away a lighted match, for it may fall on some inflammable material and thus start a fire. Never allow children to play with matches. Reading in bed by the light of a candle or lamp is likely to result in setting the bed clothing on fire if the reader goes to sleep. Lighted lamps or candles should never be placed under shelves. Clothing hung before a fire should be watched, for as soon as it is dry it may ignite. The clothing of women and children is very apt to catch fire if they lean over an open fireplace. Hot ashes put in wooden boxes or barrels are responsible for many fires.

Putting out Fires.

In cities, of course, this is generally left to a paid fire department, but if one preserves his coolness and presence of mind when he discovers a fire the fire department may find nothing to do when it arrives. Naturally, it should always be called promptly as soon as a fire is discovered. Immediately one finds a house is on fire he should go to the burning room and try to smother the fire. At first this may be accomplished by a few buckets of water or by throwing blankets or woolen clothing upon it. Sand, ashes or dirt will all quickly smother a fire. One of these should always be used instead of water on burning oil as water will spread the oil and the fire. Burning curtains or hangings should be pulled down before attempting to smother the fire in them. On the arrival of the fire department usually the best assistance that one can give will be to keep out of the way of the firemen so as not to interfere with them in their work. If no fire department is available, however, it will be best to organize a bucket brigade which should consist of two lines of men from the nearest water supply to the fire. The men in one line pass buckets, pitchers or anything else that will hold water from one to another till the last man throws the water on the fire. He returns the buckets to the water supply by the other line.

Rescue of Persons at Fires.

If a building is discovered to be on fire, send for the fire department at once. Until it arrives be sure to keep the doors closed so as to prevent drafts. If the inmates are asleep, hammer and pound on the doors to arouse them. If it proves necessary to search the burning building, enter by a door if possible and leave a responsible person to guard it so it will not be thrown open and cause a draft. Go up to the top floor and work down, examining each room as carefully as possible. If necessary to get air while making the search, it will be best to close the door of a room, then to open a window and to stick the head out till a few good breaths can be obtained. Afterward close the window to prevent a draft. While searching through a burning house it will be best to tie a wet handkerchief or cloth over the nose and mouth. Remember that the air within six inches of the floor is free from smoke, so when unable to breathe crawl along the floor with the head low, dragging anyone you have rescued behind you. Crawl backward in the same way down the staircases. Do not jump from a window unless you are compelled to and if anyone else is compelled to jump from a burning building and you are outside, put bedding and other soft substances in a pile to break the jumper's fall, or get a strong carpet or rug to catch him and have it firmly held by as many men as can secure handholds. Fire escapes will often prevent jumping, which is always dangerous, and the residents of a high building should always know how to make use of the fire escapes.

Extinguishing Burning Clothing.

If your own clothing catches on fire when you are alone, do not run for help as this will fan the flames and make them burn fiercer.

Lie down on the floor and roll up as tightly as possible in a rug, shawl, overcoat, blanket or other woolen cloth, leaving only the head out. In a bedroom one should roll up tightly in the bed clothes. If nothing can be obtained in which to wrap up, lie down and roll over slowly, at the same time beat out the fire with the hands. If another person's clothing catches fire, throw him to the ground and smother the fire with a coat, blanket, rug or the like.

Preventing Burns and Scalds from Hot Stoves, Cooking Utensils, etc.

Slight burns and scalds are, of course, not infrequent in cooks and other persons who work constantly near hot stoves. Their prevention is equally, of course, a matter of more care and attention. It is always very dangerous to allow children to play near hot stoves and as results of this practice many deaths occur annually and many children are disfigured for life.

Avoidance of Danger from Hot or Molten Metal.

Naturally, only persons working about them are subject to burns from these sources. Common care and watchfulness will do much to prevent them.

Methods to Prevent Explosions of Gas and Gunpowder.

The mixture of illuminating gas and air in certain proportions is a very explosive one. Leaky gas fixtures demand immediate attention. In case a room is entered which is filled with gas which has escaped, the door should be thrown widely open and a rush should be made to open the windows, holding the breath meanwhile, if possible. You should then leave the room and close the door till by opening it you find that the smell of gas has fairly well disappeared, when it may be entered in safety with a light.

In handling gunpowder it will be best to have no matches in
the pockets and cigars, cigarettes, pipes and lights of every description are, of course, extremely dangerous.

Symptoms of Burns and Scalds.

Severe burning pain.   Depending on depth of injury:
Reddening of skin; formation of blisters, or destruction
of the skin and some of the tissues beneath it.
Shock.

Treatment.

When the skin is simply reddened:

Exclude air by a thin paste made with water and bicarbonate of soda (baking, not washing soda), starch or
flour.   Ordinary vaselin or carbolized vaselin, olive
or castor oil, and fresh lard or cream are all good.   One
of the substances mentioned should be smeared over the
burned part and on a cloth used to cover it.   A light
bandage should be put on to hold this dressing in place.
The services of a doctor will hardly be required for such
injuries.
When blisters have formed:

Treatment may be the same, but if the blistering is very
extensive it will be best to show this injury to a doctor.
Destruction of the skin and some of the tissues beneath it:

Deep burns require prompt attention from a physician.
Pending his arrival they may be treated by the application
of the dressing which has been described or like an open
wound.
Treat shock.

Besides the burns which have been described, burns are frequently caused by strong acid and alkalies.

These injuries are sometimes due to mistaking one bottle for another. As stated under the head of Poisons, all bottles should be carefully and correctly labeled and unlabeled bottles should be thrown away. It seems almost superfluous to call attention to the necessity of keeping children away from strong acid and alkalies.

The symptoms of burns by acids and alkalies are the same as of burns caused by heat.

Treatment.

With either, wash off as quickly as possible; best under a water tap.

Acids: While washing injury, have lime-water procured or make a mixture of baking soda and water or get soapsuds and apply freely. If acid has entered the eye, wash it as quickly as possible with water and then with lime-water.

Alkalies: Wash in same way as with acid burns. Neutralize with vinegar, lemon juice or hard cider. Lime burns of the eye should be washed out with a weak solution of vinegar and water or with olive oil.

With both acid and alkali burns, after neutralizing, treat like other burns.

In severe burns of this character always see a doctor, and when either acid or alkali has entered the eye secure the services of a doctor as soon as possible.

Treat shock.

Warning.

In all burns, whatever the cause, use care in removing the clothing. When the clothing sticks to a burn, do not drag it off, cut around the part that sticks and soak it off later with oil.

5. UNCONSCIOUSNESS FROM VARIOUS CAUSES.

Unconsciousness, of course, means lack of consciousness or, in other words, one who is unconscious knows nothing of his surroundings or of what is occurring. Perhaps no condition which the first-aid student may be called upon to treat may prove more puzzling than this. Unconsciousness may result from a number of different causes, so in order to give the proper treatment one must determine first what has caused his patient to become unconscious.

Always make an earnest effort to do this by taking the surroundings into account as well as by examination of the patient.

Suppose, however, that you are unable to determine the cause of unconsciousness. At least make very sure that it is due neither to a poison, to bleeding nor to sunstroke, for each of these demands immediate special treatment. Then, unless it is necessary to give the special treatment, if the patient is pale and weak have him lie down with his head low and warm and stimulate him in every possible way; on the contrary, if the face is red and pulse is bounding and very strong, while the position for the patient should also be lying down, the head should be raised. No stimulants should be given in the latter condition and cold water should be sprinkled on face and chest.

The common causes of unconsciousness are fainting, shock, apoplexy and injury to brain, alcoholic intoxication, poisoning by opium or by some mixture containing opium, gas poisoning, carbolic acid, sunstroke, freezing, electric shock, epilepsy, hysteria, convulsions in children and uremic poisoning.

As the four last are all accompanied with convulsions, it will be more convenient to discuss them under the next heading: Fits or Convulsions.

Fainting.

Cause.

A lack of blood to the brain. Some persons, especially women, often faint.

Fainting is common in any form of weakness, as when recovering from a severe illness. Some people faint at the sight of blood.

Prevention.

A person who has not yet recovered his full strength after an illness or injury should be careful not to overdo physically. Persons who faint from trivial causes require the advice and treatment of a physician. Remember that fainting may be due to a hemorrhage, and if there is any reason to suspect that the patient is bleeding, examine him carefully and check the bleeding promptly.

Symptoms.

Usually occurs in overheated, crowded room.

Patient becomes paler and paler and finally sinks to the floor unconscious.

Unconsciousness is partial or complete.

Face is pale, frequently covered with cold perspiration.

Pupils are natural.

Breathing is shallow and sighing.

Pulse is weak and rapid.

No other cause for unconsciousness.

Treatment.

Sometimes can prevent fainting by having person who feels faint double over so that head is between knees. If this does not prove effective at once do not continue.

Air, especially cold air, and cold water often prevent actual fainting when a person feels faint.

If patient has actually fainted, put him in lying-down

position with his head lower than the rest of his body, so that brain will receive more blood. Loosen clothing, especially around neck, for same purpose. Open windows, if necessary, and keep away crowd so that patient may get plenty of air. Sprinkle face and chest with cold water. Smelling salts or ammonia to nose. Rub limbs toward body. Do not allow patient to get up until fully recovered. May give stimulant when patient has so far recovered that he is able to swallow.

Shock.

Cause.

An injury.

Prevention

Of injury.

Symptoms.

The history and probably the presence of an injury
The symptoms given under the heading Shock.

Treatment.

As given.

Apoplexy and Injury to Brain.

Apoplexy is due to the bursting of a diseased blood-vessel in the brain. The escaping blood presses on the nerve-centres and this causes the symptoms. An injury of the brain also injures these centres, so from a first-aid stand-point the symptoms and treatment of apoplexy and brain injuries may be considered under one head. Methods for preventing apoplexy are far too complicated for discussion here and, naturally, brain injuries are prevented like other injuries.

Symptoms.

Apoplexy often comes on suddenly.

In brain injury, may be history and evidence of injury to head.

In brain injury there may be hemorrhages from nose, ears, mouth and eyes.

Unconsciousness, complete.

Face: Red in apoplexy. Pale in injury.

Pupils, large and frequently unequal in size.

Eye-balls insensitive to touch.

Breathing, snoring.

Pulse: full and unusually slow.

Paralysis usually on one side of body. Test by raising arm or leg. If paralyzed, will drop absolutely helpless.

Treatment.

Send for doctor at once.

Rest and quiet, in a dark room if possible.

In lying-down position with head and shoulders high on pillows.

Ice or cold cloths to head. Hot bottles to limbs.

No stimulants.

Alcoholic Intoxication.

This represents the final stage in acute drunkenness; that is, the common spree.

Methods of prevention are clear without being discussed.

Symptoms.

Perhaps history of intoxication.

Unconsciousness, partial or complete; are frequently able to arouse patient to some extent.

Face usually flushed and bloated, but sometimes pale.

Skin cool and may be moist.

Pupils natural or large.   Eye-balls red, but not insensi-
tive to touch.
Breathing about as usual when in deep sleep.
Pulse, usually rapid and weak, but may be slow.
May be strong odor of liquor.
No paralysis.

Warning.

In practice insensibility from alcohol and apoplexy are
more often mistaken one for the other than are any other
forms of unconsciousness. The most important symptoms in which they differ are the state of the pupils, the
sensitiveness of the eye-balls and paralysis. The odor of
liquor on the breath is of no value, because a person with
apoplexy may have been drinking.

Treatment.

If any doubt whether drunkenness or apoplexy, always
treat for apoplexy and be particularly careful not to make
patient vomit, as this will cause more bleeding into brain.
In drunkenness, if able to arouse sufficiently, give
emetic—mustard and water or luke-warm water are
usually easily procured.
Afterward strong coffee or aromatic spirits of ammonia.
Hot bottles around patient.
Rub toward body to increase circulation.
Should send for doctor, as may prove dangerous.

Poisoning by Opium or by Some Mixture Containing Opium.

This is discussed at some length under Poisons.

Symptoms.

May get history of having taken opium or may find bottle
which contained poison.

Unconsciousness which comes on gradually and finally becomes complete.

Face red at first, finally dark purple. Lips bluish.

Pupils very small, like pin heads.

Breathing full and slow at first, gradually slower and shallow.

Pulse, slow and full, afterward weak.

Possibly smell of laudanum on breath.

Symptoms that should be specially noted are pin-head pupils, character of breathing and patient is first very sleepy and then becomes unconscious.

Gas Poisoning.

Poisoning by illuminating gas or by coal gas, especially from a stove or furnace, is not uncommon.

Cause.

Gas, which produces suffocation.

Prevention.

Leaks in gas pipes should be promptly repaired. Be careful in turning off gas to make sure that gas is actually shut off.

It is dangerous to leave a gas jet burning faintly when you go to sleep, as it may go out if pressure in gas main becomes less, and if pressure is afterward increased, gas may escape into room in large amount.

Coal gas will escape through red-hot cast iron, and very big fires in such stoves are dangerous, especially in sleeping rooms.

Charcoal burned in open vessels in tight rooms is especially dangerous.

Symptoms.

History of escaping gas.

First, headache, dizziness, throbbing of head, ringing in ears, spots before eyes, then gradually unconsciousness.

Face and lips bluish.

Skin pale or bluish.

Pulse weak and rapid.

Breathing intermittent.

Treatment.

Send some one else for a doctor at once.

Rescue patient promptly and bring him to room or other place where there is plenty of good air. To rescue an unconscious person in a room filled with illuminating gas, move quickly and carry him out without breathing yourself. Take a few deep breaths before entering room and hold breath while in room. If you cannot carry or drag patient from room, throw open all doors and windows and get assistance to move patient.

Loosen clothing about chest and abdomen.

Perform artificial respiration (see page 164), sprinkle cold water on face and chest, give stimulants as soon as patient recovers sufficiently to swallow.

Carbolic Acid Poisoning.

This is also discussed under Poisons.

Symptoms.

History of poison or presence of bottle which contained poison.

Vomiting and great pain.

Skin covered with cold sweat.

If severe case, unconsciousness, usually followed promptly by death.

May almost always know by the strong smell of carbolic
acid.

Lips, tongue and mouth are burned white by pure, and
black by impure carbolic acid.

Sunstroke.

This is discussed at length on page 123.

Symptoms.

Take into consideration time of year and temperature.

Unconsciousness, complete.

Face pale, red or purplish.

Skin, burning hot.

Pupils, usually small.

Breathing, slow or rapid, with more or less sighing.

Pulse, slow and full, or rapid and weak.

Freezing.

Is also discussed under proper heading.

Symptoms.

By taking into consideration the circumstances under
which patient is found, there should be no difficulty in
making out what is the matter with him.

Electric Shock.

What has been said above applies equally to electric shock
whether caused by a live wire or lightning. This condition is
also discussed under its own heading.

6. FITS OR CONVULSIONS.

Epilepsy.

This is a disease in which from time to time the patient has attacks
which are called epileptic fits. In these fits he becomes unconscious
and has convulsive movements usually of all the muscles of the body.

Cause and prevention cannot be discussed here.

Symptoms.

May be history of previous attacks.

Patient suddenly falls unconscious, with stiff and rigid muscles.

He may give a sharp cry at the beginning of a fit.

This is followed by convulsions in which the patient's whole body twitches violently and is thrown into contortions.

Foaming at the mouth is frequent and the tongue is often bitten.

After convulsions have lasted a few moments, patient may become conscious, may be confused for a time or may go into a deep sleep which will last for several hours.

There should be little difficulty in recognizing an epileptic fit.

Treatment.

Put patient where he cannot hurt himself. Best on the floor so that he can turn about without striking anything. Loosen tight clothing.

Do not try to restrain movements and do not give anything to drink.

A wad of cloth thrust in the mouth will help to prevent biting the tongue.

When patient has gone to sleep do not disturb him.

The services of a doctor are required only when convulsions are very violent and serious injury to patient appears probable.

Hysteria.

This is a nervous disease in which fits occur from time to time. It is much commoner in women than in men.

Discussion of cause and prevention would be out of place here further than to say that too much sympathy is not a kindness with hysterical people, as it makes them worse instead of better.

Symptoms.

History of previous attacks.

Usually begins with crying, sobbing or laughing without any cause or a very slight one.

Then jerky movement of limbs.

Breathing is quickened and the eyes are closed.

Patient falls to ground, taking care not to hurt herself, and becomes apparently unconscious, though not actually so.

Treatment.

Do nothing except prevent friends from sympathizing. Recovery is prompt when patient finds that her condition alarms no one.

Convulsions in Children.

The nervous system in children is affected by many causes so slight that they would have no effect in grown persons. Disturbances of the nervous system in children often result in convulsions.

Causes.

Indigestion, teething, worms, constipation, brain disease and very often in fever, especially at the beginning.

Prevention.

Consists of treatment by a doctor of one of the diseases mentioned.

Symptoms.

Usually fretful before a fit.

In fit, body is stiff, complete loss of consciousness.

Skin, wet and clammy.

Breathing, rapid.

Pulse, weak and rapid.

8

Stiffness of body is followed by jerkings and twitchings of muscles of face and body.

May be convulsion after convulsion or child may pass into a semiconscious condition and then into a deep sleep.

Treatment.

Send for doctor at once, but do not await his arrival. Convulsions in children are caused by too much blood in the brain, therefore:

Put child in hot bath for 10 to 20 minutes or give hot mustard foot-bath. At the same time apply cold to the head and neck by sponges or cloths soaked in cold water and frequently changed.

Uremic Convulsions.

Such convulsions are one of the symptoms of Bright's Disease, being due to the failure of the diseased kidneys to dispose of certain waste products of the body.

Symptoms.

May be impossible to distinguish from apoplexy if seen after unconsciousness has come on.

First,   Severe convulsions;

Then,   Unconsciousness.

May be able to obtain history of previous attack or of the patient having Bright's Disease.

May detect urinary odor.

Treatment.

Send for doctor at once.

Put to bed, cover well and surround with hot bottles.

7. POISONS.

Any substance taken into the body which will cause death is a poison. But only poisons which are swallowed will be considered here.

Prevention.

Poisons may be taken either with suicidal motive or accidentally. The reasons which make persons desire to kill themselves are so various that prevention of this cause of poisoning cannot be discussed here. On the other hand, a great deal can be said in reference to prevention of accidental poisoning.

Poisons should only be found in the household when they are urgently needed for immediate use. They should best be locked up by themselves and no one except grown members of the family should be permitted to have the keys of the boxes or cabinets in which they are locked. All poisons should be carefully labeled. Bottles from which the labels have been lost should be thrown away.

Poisoning due to decayed or spoiled food may be prevented by never using food which has begun to decay.

In opening a can of food it is always best, when possible, to use the contents of the can at once. If this is not done, the food should be immediately taken from the can and placed in a refrigerator on a clean dish.

Symptoms and Evidences of Poisoning.

The symptoms vary with the special poison. But there are certain evidences which indicate, in the majority of cases, that a poison has been taken.

Sudden and severe sickness in a person who has been in good health, after eating, drinking or taking medicine. Possibly the patient has been melancholy or has talked of suicide.

The presence near the patient of bottles, glasses or the like in which some of the poison remains.

Frequently a person who has taken poison intentionally

becomes frightened and is only too glad to tell some one that he has poisoned himself and what poison he has used.

In accidental poisoning the patient is, of course, willing to tell all he knows in reference to the poison.

If a number of persons who have eaten the same food become seriously ill after a meal, it is almost certain they are suffering from poison, probably decayed food or the so-called ptomaine poisoning.

Treatment.

The general principles to be followed in the treatment of poisoning are four in number.

1. Rid the system of the poison.

2. Neutralize it, if possible, with an antidote.

3. Stimulate patient so he can throw off its effects.

4. Soothe the digestive organs which have been irritated by it.

Send for a doctor at once and, if possible, have messenger tell him what poison has been taken so that he may bring the proper antidote.

Do not wait for doctor to arrive, but give an emetic to rid body of poison. (Some exceptions.)

Good emetics are:—

Mustard and water, salt and water, luke-warm water alone in large quantities, ipecac. The doses of each are given under the heading Emetics. Do not waste time in getting the exact dose, however, and repeat if profuse vomiting does not result.

Emetics should always be given, and at once, except with what are called corrosive poisons, which are irritating poisons which eat the parts with which they come in contact. They must, therefore, be neutralized to prevent

them eating more deeply, and with some an emetic would
be dangerous, as it would strain tissues already weakened
by the corrosive. The corrosives are the strong acids
and the strong alkalies. They often stain or burn the
hands, lips or mouth.

Corrosive sublimate and nitrate of silver are best neutralized before an emetic is given, as it is possible that a
dangerous amount may be absorbed if you wait for an
emetic to act before giving the proper antidote.

If the poison is unknown, always give an emetic at once.

If patient is weak from effects of poison and fright, give
stimulants freely—strong tea, coffee, whisky, brandy—
and cover warmly after ridding the system of the poison
or neutralizing it.

With poisons which are irritating give a soothing liquid
as well as a stimulant. Milk, raw eggs beaten up or
flour and water, all serve this purpose.

The subject of poisoning usually proves more difficult than any
other for the student of first aid.

The table which follows is given to assist him to remember or to
call to mind the symptoms and treatment of the common poisons.

TABLE I.

Poisons.

With which an emetic is always given first.

Poison	Symptoms	Treatment (besides emetic)
Unknown.		Stimulants, soothing liquids.
Alcohol: In any form—rum, gin, whisky, p r o o f s p i r i t s, etc., also methyl alcohol.	Giddiness, swaying of body, i n a b i l i t y to stand. Face flushed, eyes red, skin clammy, weak pulse, may be convulsions and unconsciousness.	Hot coffee or aromatic spirits of ammonia. Try to arouse, but if weak do not exhaust by m a k i n g w a l k. Dash cold water on face and chest. When somewhat recovered, wrap warmly and put to bed.
Arsenic: Found in rat poisons, vermin killer, Paris green, Fowler's solution. Sometimes in tinned f r u i t s a n d beer.	Severe pain in stomach, purging, severe cramps in legs, vomiting, d r y n e s s of throat, c o l d sweats, profound shock.	Much luke-warm water. Magnesia in l a r g e quantity or dialyzed iron in $\frac{1}{2}$-oz. doses, repeated. B e a t e n up eggs or castor oil and stimulants. Warmth and rubbing. If rat poison has been taken, treat as for poisoning by arsenic.
Lead: Sugar of lead, lead paint, white lead.	Throat d r y, metallic taste with much thirst, colic in abdomen, cramps in legs, cold sweat. Sometimes paralysis of legs and convulsions.	$\frac{1}{2}$ oz. epsom salts in tumbler of water. Stimulants and soothing liquids.

Poison	Symptoms	Treatment (besides emetic)
Opium: Laudanum, morphin, paregoric, some soothing syrups and cough mixtures.	Drowsiness, finally unconsciousness. Pulse full at first, then weak, breathing full and slow at first, gradually slower and shallow, pin-head pupils, face flushed, then purple.	May have difficulty in getting emetic to work. Plenty of strong coffee. Try to arouse by speaking loudly and threatening, but do not exhaust by compelling to walk, etc. Stimulants and artificial respiration.
Phosphorus: In matches, phosphorus paste in many rat poisons and vermin killers, often with arsenic.	Severe pain in stomach, vomiting. Skin is dark and may have odor of phosphorus. Bleeding from nose, bloody purging. Convulsions.	Epsom salts, $\frac{1}{2}$ oz., in tumbler of water, or magnesia. Stimulants. Soothing liquid best. Milk. Avoid fats and oils.
Ptomaine: Poisoning by decayed meat, fish, milk or ice cream.	Nausea, vomiting, purging. Skin cold and clammy. Pulse weak. Severe pain in abdomen, cramps, great prostration and weakness. Often eruption on skin	Purgative, castor oil or epsom salts. Teaspoonful of powdered charcoal and repeat.
Strychnine— Nux Vomica: Strychnine is frequently used on meat to poison animals and in some vermin killers.	Convulsions, very severe, alternating with cramps, affecting all muscles of body. Back is bowed up by spasms of muscles. Jaws are locked. Spasm of muscles is so great that prevents breathing, so face becomes dusky.	Powdered charcoal, if possible in large quantity. Follow with another emetic. Absolute quiet so as not to bring on convulsions.

TABLE II.

Poisons.

For which an emetic should not be given first.

Poison	Symptoms	Treatment
Mercury: Corrosive sublimate, antiseptic tablets. Other salts of mercury much less commonly used.	*Corrosive sublimate is very irritating so when taken turns mouth, lips and tongue white. Mouth is swollen and tongue is shriveled; always metallic taste in mouth. Pain in abdomen. Nausea and vomiting mucus and blood, bloody purging, cold clammy skin, great prostration and convulsions.	First, give white of egg or whole egg beating it up. Flour and water, but not so good. Emetics, soothing liquids and stimulants.
Nitrate of silver: Lunar caustic.	Pain in mouth and stomach. Mouth first colored white, then black. Vomit first white, then turns black.	Common salt dissolved in water, or milk very frequently. Then emetic. Afterward, soothing liquids and stimulants.

TABLE III.

Poisons.

With which an emetic should not be given.

Poison	Symptoms	Treatment
Strong corrosive acids: 1. Acetic. 2. Hydrochloric (Spirits of salt) 3. Nitric (Aqua fortis). 4. Sulphuric (Vitriol).	Very severe burning pain in mouth, throat and stomach. Wherever acid touches skin or mucous membrane they are destroyed. Frequently vomiting and purging. More or less suffocation from swelling of throat, great prostration and shock.	An alkali to neutralize acid. Best, magnesia or chalk in water given frequently and freely. Lime, whiting, baking soda, plaster, tooth powder or even wood ashes may all be used for alkali, or ammonia, a tablespoonful to two cups of water, but those mentioned above are better as they are less irritating. Afterward, soothing liquids, milk; milk and egg, olive oil. Stimulants are practically always required. If acid has entered air-passage, may inhale fumes of ammonia.
Oxalic acid: (Salts of lemon or sorrel).	Much like corrosive acids just named, but not so much burning of lips, etc.	Magnesia, chalk and water or lime-water to neutralize acid. Then 1 oz. of castor oil and stimulants freely.

Poison	Symptoms	Treatment
Carbolic acid (phenol): (Very commonly used in attempts at suicide.)	Is also a powerful corrosive poison which causes great pain and vomiting. Severe; unconsciousness, very soon and early death. Usually easy to tell by odor of acid and burn, which with pure acid is white, and with impure, black.	Rinse mouth with pure alcohol. If grown person, should swallow 3 or 4 tablespoonfuls of alcohol mixed with an equal quantity of water. Follow this in 5 minutes with 2 tablespoonfuls of epsom salts dissolved in a little water. Though not so good, lime-water may be used to rinse mouth, several glasses of it being also swallowed. Three or four raw eggs may be given or castor or sweet oil. Stimulants always, and keep warm.
Strong caustic alkalies: 1. Ammonia: Strong ammonia. Ammonia liniment. Camphor liniment. 2. Lime: Quicklime. 3. Potash: Caustic potash. 4. Soda: Caustic soda.	Much like corrosive acids. Immediate severe burning, pain in mouth, throat and stomach. Vomiting and purging. Alkali destroys tissues of mouth it has touched. Severe shock and suffocation from swelling.	An acid to neutralize alkali. Vinegar, lemon or orange juice. Tartaric or citric acid in plenty of water. Soothing liquids, stimulants. If cannot swallow may inhale acetic acid or vinegar from a pocket handkerchief.

Caution:

In giving any antidote, do not wait for it to dissolve, but stir it up in any fluid which can be obtained except oil, and give at once.

8. SUNSTROKE AND HEAT EXHAUSTION.

Sunstroke.

This is a condition produced by excessive heat. It is a very dangerous one.

Cause.

Sometimes due to direct exposure to the rays of the hot summer sun, especially when the air is moist.

Most commonly due, however, to somewhat prolonged exposure to excessive heat while working indoors, especially if overfatigued.

Too heavy clothing is likely to help to cause sunstroke, and hats and caps which do not protect the head from the sun are dangerous.

Drinking any kind of alcoholic liquor before physical exertion with exposure to the summer sun is very apt to result in sunstroke.

Prevention.

Avoidance of exposure to sun in middle of day in summer. The best possible ventilation of workrooms in summer, and avoidance of over-fatigue as far as possible.

Light clothing for summer and light head-gear with space above head for ventilation. Preferably head-gear should have orange-red lining.

Avoid alcohol before exposure to sun.

If one feels the first symptoms of sunstroke he can often prevent actual sunstroke by stopping work, finding a cool place, lying down, bathing face, hands and chest in cold water and drinking freely of cold water.

Symptoms.

Usually before actual attack, pain in head and feeling of oppression.

Unconsciousness complete.
Face red.
Pupils dilated.
Skin very hot and dry.
No perspiration.
Breathing labored and sighing.
Pulse slow and full.

Treatment.

Consists in reducing temperature.
Send for doctor.
Remove at once to cool place.
Loosen and remove as much clothing as possible.
Apply cold to head and body. To do this, cold water or ice should be rubbed over face, neck, chest and in armpits. Is still better to put patient in a very cold bath or to wrap him in sheets wrung out in cold water which should be kept wet and cold with water or ice. If this is done, must rub continually to prevent shock and to bring hot blood to surface.
When consciousness returns, may be allowed to drink cold water freely.
Cold may be discontinued when consciousness returns, but if skin again becomes very hot, must renew.
No stimulants.

Heat Exhaustion.

Though this condition is caused and prevented in the same ways as sunstroke, it is really quite different from it. Heat exhaustion is just what its name states—exhaustion or collapse due to excessive heat.

Symptoms.

Great depression and weakness.

No unconsciousness.

Face pale and covered with clammy sweat.

Breathing shallow.

Pulse weak and rapid.

Treatment.

Send for doctor.

Remove to cool place and have patient lie down in most comfortable position with clothing loosened.

No cold externally, but may sip cold water.

Stimulants, as tea, coffee, aromatic spirits of ammonia or small amount of brandy or whisky with a good deal of water.

9. FROST-BITE AND FREEZING.

Frost-bite.

This is due to the local effect of cold on the body, parts of which freeze much as do certain other objects. The parts of the body which are most liable to frost-bite are the nose, ears, toes and fingers.

Cause.

Cold; insufficient clothing; general weakness with poor circulation of blood.

Prevention.

Protection of the body, especially the exposed parts named above with sufficient covering when it is necessary to expose yourself to intense cold.

Rubbing of any part of the body which becomes very cold in order to increase circulation.

Symptoms.

In intense cold, frost-bite not infrequently occurs without one knowing it, but usually the ears, fingers, etc., become painfully cold and then one suddenly realizes that they no longer have feeling.

The color of the frozen part is white or grayish-white.

Treatment.

Object: To gradually bring the frozen part to its natural temperature.

Rub with snow or cold water. Then warm the water gradually.

Warning.

The use of heat at once may result in mortification or death of the frozen part.

Freezing.

This condition is produced by long exposure to extreme cold.

Cause.

Extreme cold.

Effect of which is increased by overexertion, hunger, alcoholic liquors and insufficient clothing.

Prevention.

If you expect to be exposed to extreme cold, procure warm clothing sufficient in amount to protect you from its effects. Do not attempt a long journey in the cold without food and do not make the journey so long that you are likely to have to stop and perhaps lie down on account of exhaustion. Do not drink alcoholic liquors, for though they give a temporary sense of warmth, you will be easily overcome by cold after this effect wears off.

If caught out without shelter in very cold weather use all your energy to keep moving. Lying down under such circumstances almost always results in freezing.

Symptoms.

Circumstances should be taken into account. Depression is so great that appearance of patient is like that of a dead man.

Treatment.

Object is gradually to restore warmth to the body.

Take patient into a cold room, rub limbs toward body with rough clothes wet in cool water, increase temperature of room if possible. This should be done gradually and clothes should be wet in warmer and warmer water. As soon as patient can swallow, give stimulant—coffee or tea in small quantities, frequently repeated with the addition of a little whisky or brandy.

Patient should not be placed before an open fire or in a hot bath until circulation has become active in cool room. You will know this by an increased force of the pulse, better breathing and more warmth and color in the skin.

10. ELECTRICITY AND LIGHTNING STROKE.

Electricity.

The more general use of electricity is making accidents due to it more common year by year. Even now the third rail and the live wire are responsible for many injuries and deaths.

The ordinary trolley wire carries a current of about 500 volts and incandescent and arc-light currents run from 2500 to 3000 volts. The passage of these powerful currents through the body causes dangerous shock or even death.

Prevention.

The third rail is always dangerous, so avoid it.

Swinging wires of any kind may somewhere in their course be in contact with live wires, so they should not be touched.

Symptoms.

Sudden loss of consciousness when the electrical current passes through the body.

Shallow breathing and weak pulse.

If hands are in contact with a live wire, person may not be able to release them at first.

Burns of hands or other parts of the body are common. Little difficulty should be experienced in making out cause of injury.

Treatment.

First, rescue; second, treat patient.

Rescue.

Patient in contact with wire or rail carrying an electric current will transfer current to rescuer if he puts himself in the line of passage of the current.

Therefore, he must not touch the body of a person suffering from electric shock still touching a live wire or a third rail unless his own body is thoroughly insulated. Naturally, too, he must not himself, in attempting to aid the injured person, bring any part of his own body in contact with the live wire or other apparatus carrying the electric current. Moreover, he must act very promptly for the danger to the patient is much increased the longer the electrical current is permitted to pass through his body. If possible, the rescuer should insulate himself by covering his hands with a mackintosh, rubber sheeting, several thicknesses of silk, or even of dry cloth. In addition he should, if possible, complete his insulation by standing on a dry board or a thick piece of dry paper, or even on a dry coat. Rubber gloves and shoes or boots are still safer, but they cannot usually be procured quickly. If a live wire is under a patient and the ground is dry it will be perfectly safe to stand upon it and to pull him off the wire with the bare hands. But they should touch only his clothing and this must not be wet.

A live wire lying on a patient may with safety be flipped off with a dry board or stick.

In removing the live wire from the patient, or the patient from the wire, do this with one motion as rocking him to and fro on the wire will increase shock and burn.

A live wire may be safely cut by an axe or hatchet with a dry wooden handle and the electrical current may be short-circuited by dropping a crowbar or poker on the wire. Drop the metal bar, do not place it on the wire or you will then be made a part of the short circuit and receive the current of electricity through your body.

How to treat Patient as soon as he has been Rescued.

Send for a doctor.

Loosen clothing around neck, chest and abdomen. Perform artificial respiration for at least 30 minutes if he does not breathe earlier without it. Stimulants as soon as patient can swallow. Keep him as warm as possible. Prompt treatment, especially artificial respiration carried on for a considerable time, will result in the recovery of most patients unless the shock has been immediately fatal.

Lightning Stroke.

Lightning produces the effect of a very powerful current of electricity.

The prevention of lightning stroke cannot be stated accurately as lightning is subject to so many freaks. During a thunder storm, however, persons exposed on a flat plain or under a large tree are probably in more danger than in a house.

9

The fear of being struck by lightning is not well grounded, as injuries from this cause are relatively very uncommon.

Symptoms.

Same as from a powerful electrical shock.

Death is not infrequent. If this does not occur, unconsciousness with great depression is usual.

Burns, also commonly result from lightning.

Treatment.

Same as for shock from an electrical current.

Burns from any form of electricity are treated like other burns.

EMERGENCY SUPPLIES.

In England, the St. John's Ambulance Association has provided boxes of emergency supplies which are placed at convenient points on the streets of cities. Nothing of this kind is available in our country, so for such supplies we must rely on what we can find at hand or make and on what we can get from drug stores.

The supplies required for each of the common accidents and injuries have been given in the preceding pages and need not be repeated. It is well to remember, however, that in treating any accident or injury you must determine promptly what supplies you will need. Often some of them may be gotten from by-standers. Naturally, the others must be sent for. As a general rule, do not leave your patient but send someone else who has not your knowledge of first aid to get the supplies you need. Try to explain to him clearly just what you want and if you know, tell him where to go. If you send him to a drug store it will be best, in order to avoid mistakes, to give him a list which he may hand to the druggist.

At the end of the next chapter will be found a list of supplies which should commonly be kept on hand at home, and under "Camping," a list of those required in far away places.

The contents of the first-aid box of the St. John's Ambulance Association, slightly changed here on account of national differences, are as follows:

1 Set wooden splints, 2 tourniquets, 1 package bichloride gauze, 1 package absorbent cotton, 3 U. S. Army first-aid dressings, 12 roller bandages, gauze, assorted sizes; 6 triangular bandages, 1 pair scissors, 1 knife, 1 graduate, 2 oz. each olive oil and aromatic spirits of ammonia, 4 oz. carbolized vaseline, pins, safety pins, needles and thread.

CHAPTER VII.

COMMON EMERGENCIES.

1. Cramp or Colic. 2. Diarrhea. 3. Constipation. 4. Vomiting. 5. Hiccough. 6. Chill from Exposure. 7. Nervous Attacks. 8. Croup. 9. Neuralgia of Face. 10. Tooth-ache. 11. Ear-ache. 12 Styes. 13. Prickly Heat. 14. Chilblains. 15. Corns. Emergency Supplies for the Home.

1. CRAMP OR COLIC.

This condition is such a common one that it is almost unnecessary to describe it. As everybody knows, abdominal cramp is a severe pain in the abdomen which is not constant. The cramps may follow one another very rapidly or there may be some time between them.

Cause.

As has been explained under the head of anatomy there are a number of different structures in the abdomen. The common cramp is due to a spasm of the intestines caused by indigestible food, or by cold, especially when overheated in hot weather. More uncommon causes are appendicitis and gall or kidney stones.

Prevention.

As one of the commonest causes of cramp is indigestible food you should be careful to avoid this; unripe fruit and partially spoiled food are most dangerous. Even in very hot weather the abdomen should be lightly covered,

132

especially at night, and if one is subject to cramps they will
often be prevented by the use of an abdominal band.
Prevention of cramp due to the other causes which have
been mentioned is too complicated a subject for discussion
except in medical books.

Symptoms.

Severe cramping pain in the abdomen and shock in
severe cases. If shock is severe, it is well to conclude that
something more serious than intestinal cramp is present.

Treatment.

A hot bottle placed on the abdomen or rubbing it will
often give relief. Soda mint tablets, or even better, hot
water with a little spirits of peppermint or syrup of ginger
should be taken. Indigestible matter may be gotten rid
of by vomiting or by a cathartic, such as a compound
cathartic pill, salts, or a Seidlitz powder. If shock is
severe always send for a doctor.

2. DIARRHEA.

Is caused just as is the common type of abdominal cramp and
naturally its prevention is the same.

Treatment.

The object of treatment is to expel the indigestible matter
from the bowels. This is best accomplished by giving
$\frac{1}{10}$-grain doses of calomel, 15 minutes apart until 6
doses are taken and by following this after 8 or 10 hours by
a Seidlitz powder or a dose of Epsom Salts.

After this if the diarrhea continues with considerable
cramping pain a teaspoonful of syrup of ginger in $\frac{1}{3}$ of a
glass of water should be given after each passage. For
painless diarrhea, 20 grains of subnitrate of bismuth, 3
times daily, is a good and safe remedy. For children a

dose of castor oil should be given instead of the remedies which have been mentioned.

The diet is also of great importance in diarrhea and nothing should be eaten which will furnish new food for fermentation or will irritate the digestive organs.

Milk in small quantities is the best food for both grown-ups and children. Boiling the milk is the wiser plan unless it is certain that it is very fresh and pure.

If the remedies mentioned do not cure the diarrhea it is much safer to consult a doctor. There are any number of so-called cholera cures on the market but the majority contain opium in some form and are therefore dangerous, especially for children.

3. CONSTIPATION.

Constipation may be prevented in most people. Persons inclined to be constipated should be careful to eat bulky food; oatmeal and the like are especially good as they irritate the intestines slightly. They should also drink plenty of water. Many persons too suffer from chronic constipation because they are careless and do not establish regular habits. Instead of always resorting to cathartics one who suffers from chronic constipation should try to get rid of the cause of this condition. To do this the advice of a doctor is required.

For acute constipation, six $\frac{1}{10}$-gr. doses of calomel at intervals of 15 minutes, taken at night and a Seidlitz Powder or a dose of Epsom Salts the next morning are excellent remedies.

4. NAUSEA AND VOMITING.

These are also usually due to indigestible food but may be caused by dyspepsia or nervousness.

Treatment.

When due to indigestible food, several large drinks of luke warm water will usually cause free vomiting and will wash out the stomach which is very desirable. The further treatment is the same whatever the cause. Patient should lie down in cool place. Hot applications to abdomen; cloths wrung out in hot water or a mustard plaster. A soda mint tablet or a little baking soda will usually stop both nausea and vomiting and in other cases sucking small lumps of ice will be found efficacious.

5. HICCOUGH.

Is usually due to overeating and indigestion. It is caused by a spasmodic contraction of the diaphragm, the great muscle which separates the chest from the abdomen. This is the reason that holding the breath as long as possible will usually cure it as the air in the chest forces the diaphragm down so it does not contract. Drinking a large glass of water in small sips without taking a breath has exactly the same effect. The reason that a scare stops hiccough sometimes is because this causes the patient to take a long breath. If none of these methods are successful, vomiting by removing the irritating material from the stomach will almost always cure the hiccough.

6. CHILL FROM EXPOSURE.

When one is exposed to the cold, especially to cold rain or snow or falls into cold water he will often become what is commonly called "chilled through."

Cause.

This condition is due to the fact that the cold contracts the blood-vessels of the skin, driving the blood to the interior of the body. This gives one the sensation of chilliness.

Prevention.

Is, of course, sufficient clothing and avoidance of exposure to cold.

Symptoms.

The sensation of cold. The lips become blue and the teeth chatter.

Treatment.

Remove the clothing if possible, and put into a warm bed covering the patient warmly. Two or three hot bottles will warm the bed well. Rubbing his limbs and body will also bring the blood to the surface and so help to cure the chill. Hot drinks should also be given. Hot tea, hot coffee, hot milk and hot lemonade, are all good.

7. NERVOUS ATTACKS.

These are usually a mild form of hysteria, and, like hysterical fits, are more common in women. The patient usually has a fit of shivering and complains of feeling cold and upset. The treatment is exactly the same as that described for a chill from exposure.

8. CROUP.

This is a children's disease due to a spasm or contraction of the muscles of the upper air-passages. Children often have what is called a croupy cough whenever they catch cold. This is a hard ringing cough which is distressing but not particularly alarming except to parents who fear, perhaps from previous experience, that an attack of true croup is coming on. Lighting the light, talking to the child, reading to him, or telling a favorite story will often result in the attack passing off and in the child becoming drowsy and finally going to sleep.

True croup is much more alarming though not often dangerous. The child has the ringing cough and croupy crow and becomes partially suffocated because sufficient air does not enter the lungs. The face becomes bluish and the child struggles to get its breath.

Treatment.

Send for a doctor but do not wait for him to arrive. Such a child should at once be given an emetic. A teaspoonful of syrup of ipecac is best for this purpose or a ½ teaspoonful of powdered alum followed by a drink of warm water. Then cloths wrung out in as hot water as the child can stand should be put about the throat and on the chest. These should be covered with a piece of dry cloth, or better of oiled silk if this can be procured. Change these cloths as soon as they begin to grow cool, but do nothing further till the physician arrives.

9. NEURALGIA OF THE FACE.

Some people are very subject to neuralgia or pain in some of the nerves of the face. This neuralgia may be due to the irritation of a bad tooth or to some other irritation less easily found but unfortunately in certain people the cause cannot be discovered. Persons who suffer from attacks of neuralgia should always consult a doctor, but such attacks often come on suddenly when no physician can be obtained.

Treatment.

Hot applications are usually better than cold ones and should always be tried first unless the patient knows from previous experience that cold will do him more good. Either hot water, or cloths wrung out in hot or cold water may be used. Painting the painful part with the ordinary menthol stick relieves many people. Some are benefited by the irritation produced by rubbing, and pressure on the painful nerve often gives temporary relief.

If the neuralgia is due to a bad tooth the proper emergency treatment of the tooth will frequently cure the neuralgia.

10. TOOTH-ACHE.

The prevention of decay of the teeth consists in the removal of all food from between them for such food ferments quickly thus producing an acid which corrodes the teeth. The teeth should be brushed night and morning and after each meal, if possible. Dental floss should also be used if difficulty is experienced in dislodging particles from between the teeth with a brush.

As has been explained under Anatomy, tooth-ache is due to decay and to food entering a cavity of a tooth where it decomposes and causes irritation and pain of the sensitive nerves.

Treatment.

If the cavity can be reached, it should be cleaned out and afterward something put in it to deaden the nerve. To clean it, twist a very small piece of cotton around a tooth-pick or fine knitting-needle and put it in the hole in the tooth, twisting it around and around so as to clean out the cavity thoroughly. After this has been done another small piece of cotton should be dipped in oil of cloves and then gently put into the cavity on the end of the tooth-pick or needle. Tooth-wax is used in the same way. If the cavity cannot be reached, the aching tooth must be treated by an application to its gum between the latter and the cheek. A small piece of absorbent cotton soaked in spirits of camphor is excellent for this purpose. The burning caused by it is severe, but it will usually cure the tooth-ache. Tooth-plasters may be used in the same way. Of course, these are merely emergency measures, and because they cure the toothache for the time being, this does not mean that it is safe for you to go on without the services of a dentist. You should realize that unless you have proper attention, decay will go on in the tooth, you will have toothache again, and will probably finally lose the tooth.

11. EAR-ACHE.

This is particularly common in children, and may be due to bad teeth, to disease of the throat or to trouble in the ear itself.

Treatment.

The teeth should always be examined, and if a cavity is found it should be treated in the way already described. If nothing is found the matter with the teeth or treatment of bad teeth fails to relieve the pain in the ear, it will be necessary to try to stop the pain by treating the ear itself. Cloths wrung out in hot water, changed as soon as they begin to grow cold, or a hot-water bottle put on the face covering the outside of the ear will often cure ear-ache. Another method is to heat a cloth very hot and to pour a few drops of alcohol on its centre and then apply this over the ear so that the alcohol fumes will enter the ear. Alcohol on a hot shovel is even better, but harder to use. Heating sweet oil just hot enough not to burn and then putting a few drops in the ear and introducing a small plug of absorbent cotton should be tried if the other remedies mentioned do not prove effective.

Severe ear-ache always demands the services of a doctor as disease of the inner ear may result in perforation of the ear-drum, which may often be prevented by a physician if treated promptly.

12. STYES.

Styes are a local inflammation at the edge of the eye-lid, usually of the small glands there. As they commonly indicate ill health or an error in vision, a doctor should be consulted in order that he may give treatment which will prevent styes appearing again. The pain of a stye may be diminished to a considerable extent by the use of compresses as hot as can be borne. If pus appears, a doctor should make the small cut necessary to permit it to escape.

13. PRICKLY HEAT.

Is the well-known irritating disease of the skin produced by heat. It is most common in children whose skin is very delicate and occurs in hot weather, not infrequently being due in part to too much clothing. It may be prevented to a great extent, even in the tropics, by not exercising so as to produce sweating and by avoiding heating drinks. A good talcum powder frequently applied also does much to prevent this annoying affection.

When prickly heat is severe the skin should be bathed with a mixture of one part of alcohol and three of water, afterward dusting on talcum powder. Lime-water with about two drops of carbolic acid to the oz. is an excellent application for prickly heat, as the carbolic acid numbs the nerves of the irritated and painful skin.

14. CHILBLAINS.

This common condition is caused by local chilling of some part of the body and is most frequently seen in old people with poor circulation. The most common places for chilblains are the heel, toes, ears, nose and fingers.

In susceptible people, as it is due to cold, it may be prevented by warm clothing and frequent bathing of the part of the body affected in warm water, afterward drying it with soft towels.

Symptoms.

They are the well-known red appearance of the skin, which appears when the part is brought near the heat, especially in winter after being in the cold. There is considerable burning and itching.

Treatment.

Paint every two or three days with tincture of iodine pure or diluted with alcohol. Several coats of collodion at intervals of a few days are also good, as the collodion exerts considerable pressure on the dilated blood-vessels. If these measures fail, it is best to consult a physician, as chilblains are sometimes very difficult to cure.

15. CORNS.

Corns are of two kinds—hard and soft. The former occur at the sides of the toes and at the sides and bottoms of the feet. Soft corns occur between the toes where the natural secretion makes the skin soft and pulpy. Both varieties of corns may be prevented by the most scrupulous cleanliness of the feet and stockings and by wearing well-fitting shoes which do not rub and so cause irritation of the skin which leads to the formation of a corn.

If a callous begins to form, rub the place gently with vaseline night and morning. Nitrate of silver stick will usually cause corns to disappear. An excellent corn remedy is one part of salicylic acid to three parts of simple cerate. Bathe and soak the foot in hot water for twenty minutes, dry and apply ointment; cover corn with cotton.

Hard corns should never be cut, but should be rubbed down smooth with sandpaper after washing the skin. They should then be covered with a corn plaster or a piece of adhesive plaster. Cutting a corn, if you get below the hard skin of the corn, is likely to prove very dangerous, as it often results in blood-poisoning.

Soft corns should be treated by careful washing and drying of the foot, especially between the toes, then dusting in a little talcum powder and keeping the toes separated by a small piece of gauze. A corn which has become inflamed requires treatment from a doctor on account of the danger of blood-poisoning.

EMERGENCY SUPPLIES FOR THE HOME.

In every household, even in the middle of a city with drug stores near by, it is wise to have a few simple remedies and surgical dressings on hand. This is more especially the case if there are children in the household, as little people are so likely to hurt themselves and are much more liable to sudden illness than are grown-ups.

Neat emergency cases which fill all requirements fairly well may be purchased. Being specially made for the purpose, they possess the advantage of having a place for everything and everything in its place. They are rather expensive, however, and there is no reason, if you care to take the trouble, why you cannot buy your own box and fill it to suit your own particular requirements. The standard size for your bottles of liquid medicines had best be 2 ounces, and the square bottles should be used. The box should be just high enough to take a 2-ounce bottle corked, standing up, and big enough for all the supplies you need. Medicines prescribed by a doctor in illness are much better put in a safe place where they will not be meddled with, so it will be wise to leave space for them in your box. This may be made of metal or hard wood and should, preferably, have a key.

The supplies suggested for the ordinary first aid household box are as follows:

Alcohol.
Aromatic Spirits of Ammonia (rubber cork).
Castor Oil.
Epsom Salts (or $\frac{1}{2}$ doz. Seidlitz Powders).

Lime-water.

Mustard, powdered.

Sodium Bicarbonate.

Syrup of Ginger.

Syrup of Ipecac.

Witch-hazel.

$\frac{1}{10}$-grain Calomel Tablets (small bottle, 50–100 tablets).

5-gr. Bismuth Subnitrate tablets (100).

Carbolized Vaseline (1 glass jar).

1 drachm bottle Oil of Cloves (labeled "Poison").

1 bottle 50 Soda Mint Tablets.

1 Tin Talcum Powder.

1 small package antiseptic gauze.

$\frac{1}{2}$ pound Absorbent Cotton.

6 Gauze Roller Bandages (3 large and 3 small).

2 U. S. Army First Aid Dressings.

1 Roll Oiled Silk.

1 Roll old Muslin.

1 Small bottle Collodion, with brush.

1 box Tooth-wax.

1 box Tooth-plasters.

1 box Corn-plasters.

1 Sharp Knife.

1 Pair Scissors.

Pins, ordinary and safety.

CHAPTER VIII.

OCCUPATION ACCIDENTS AND INJURIES.

1. Railroad Injuries. 2. Injuries of Factory and Workshop. 3. Injuries of Farm and Ranch. 4. Mining Injuries. 5. Business Injuries. Hernia or Rupture

RAILROAD INJURIES.

The last report of the Interstate Commerce Commission shows 16,613 people killed and 97,706 injured on railways during the preceding year.

This certainly demonstrates the necessity for a knowledge of first aid on the part of railroad men. Naturally, however, they are not interested in all classes of accidents and emergencies, as some of these are not of great practical importance to them. It is suggested, therefore, that in studying this book they pay particular attention to the first three chapters, to the chapter on Transportation, to the section, Bruises to Fractures, to that on Wounds and to the present section.

Causes.

The causes of railway injuries are various: coupling cars frequently results in the crushing of the hands of brakemen; wrecks; falling from trains; being struck by cars, etc.

Prevention.

EMPLOYEES.

Proper instruction in the theory and practice of safety in railroading by the company.

144

Safety appliances provided by the company.

Common care on the part of employees.

Reasonable hours of work so that physical exhaustion does not cause indifference and carelessness; an obligation of the company.

General instruction in first aid for employees.

PASSENGERS AND OTHERS.

(Suggested by one of our most prominent railroad men.)

"Never cross a railway at a grade crossing before making sure that no trains are approaching."

"Never jump on or off cars in motion."

"Never stand on platforms of cars in motion."

"Never put head or other part of person out of car window."

"Never cross in front or rear of standing or moving train without first making sure that there is no danger from some other train or cause."

"Never disobey the cautionary rules for safety posted at stations, crossings, etc."

"Never forget that carelessness on your part in regard to these precautions not only endangers your life, but the happiness and welfare of those most dear to you."

Symptoms.

These naturally depend upon the character of the particular injury.

The commonest railway injuries are fractures and severe wounds, sometimes clean-cut, but more often lacerated with not infrequently actual tearing off of fingers and toes. Severe crushing and mangling injuries are also common and trifling wounds are a matter of every day occurrence on every railroad.

10

Wounds produced by railway injuries are usually dirty as grease and coal dust are frequently ground into them. The crushing often prevents severe hemorrhage, but, on the other hand, tissues torn apart frequently bleed freely. Shock is generally severe.

Treatment.

A railroad wreck probably emphasizes the value of a knowledge of first aid better than any other accident. Too often, excited people totally ignorant of what they should do, harm injured more than help them. In a railroad wreck every one who can do so should at first be employed in removing injured from the wrecked cars. This is especially true if there is danger from fire. The injured should be taken far enough from the wreck so that people about it will not stumble over them. If two men with a knowledge of first aid are present, one should post himself at the wreck so that he may instruct the helpers how to carry patients in order not to injure them further, and the other should take care of the patients at the place selected for them.

Railway injuries involve no principles of treatment which have not been taught in the preceding pages. Crushes when bones are broken demand the careful application of splints, and railway wounds of every sort should be treated just like other wounds. It should never be forgotten that shock is severe in this class of injuries and demands careful treatment.

Not infrequently in railroad injuries on arrival of the patient at a hospital it is found that he has lost so much blood that his condition is hopeless. Remember, therefore, to check hemorrhage as far as possible, for even if it is not immediately alarming, within a comparatively

short time if hemorrhage continues a dangerous amount
of blood will be lost. Besides shock at the time of injury
weakens the heart, which beats more strongly again
after reaction begins and then much blood may be lost
from torn vessels.

It seems quite unnecessary to call attention to the fact
that the services of a doctor are required promptly for
such injuries.

Certain emergency supplies are necessary for the treatment of railway injuries. This need has been met in
England by a special hamper which the St. John Ambulance Association has made up for railway purposes.
Its contents are practically the same as those of the first-
aid box described on page 131, though the number of
bandages and the quantity of aromatic spirits of ammonia,
especially useful for shock, have been somewhat increased.
Even a few first-aid packets and a flask of aromatic
spirits of ammonia will prove of the greatest value in
cases of need.

While the time will undoubtedly come when emergency
supplies will be found on our railway trains, or at least in
an accident room at railway centres, this is not the case at
present. We must, therefore, almost always rely on
what we can find near at hand.

Splints may be made from the canes and umbrellas of
the passengers or in a wreck from pieces of the broken
cars. Pillows may also sometimes be obtained. Unused
linen from a sleeping-car makes a much better covering
for a wound than dirty clothing. Bandages may also be
made from sheets.

For shock the patient should always be put in the lying-
down position with his head low, on a mattress if one is

obtainable. He should be well covered with blankets or coats. Shock, of course, demands the use of some stimulant, and an effort should be made to obtain some whisky from passengers or bystanders. Do not give whisky in large quantities, however. If a doctor may be expected to arrive soon, one large drink of whisky should be given; but if the patient must go several hours before he can have care from a doctor, it will be better to give him a teaspoonful of whisky in a tablespoonful of water and to repeat this every ten minutes if necessary, depending on his condition.

The injured man may be carried on a mattress or the coat litter may be used.

2. INJURIES OF FACTORY AND WORK-SHOP.

Naturally, the liability to such injuries and their kind varies greatly according to the particular work on which a person is employed. It is not necessary, however, to discuss the different injuries of this class at length, as their symptoms and treatment are exactly the same as with such injuries in general.

Injuries of the factory and work-shop are, of course, frequent, so that knowledge of first aid on the part of employees is almost, if not quite as necessary, as for railroad men. Their study may be confined to the subjects recommended for railway men. The study of Burns should also receive careful attention in certain cases. The excellent practice of sending selected employees to study first aid at the expense of the company has already been adopted by many employers.

Causes.

Being caught in machinery, cut by saws, burns from molten metal or caustics, falls, etc.

Prevention.

> Sufficient instruction to do work with reasonable safety; an obligation of the employer.
>
> Safety appliances; employer.
>
> Common care (do not risk injury or death in order to save labor and do not be reckless); employees.
>
> Knowledge of first aid; employees.

Symptoms.

> Same as with like injuries in general, but naturally vary greatly with injury.
>
> Machinery accidents produce mangling, tearing and crushing injuries not unlike railroad injuries. Power saws and other sharp instruments cause clean cuts which bleed freely. Electrical shocks are common in certain industries. In chemical works burns from caustics are frequent and in foundries and rolling mills burns due to contact with molten metal are equally common.
>
> Shock is generally severe with all these injuries.

Treatment.

> As with injuries in general, do not forget to treat shock.
>
> The first-aid box described on page 131 or a box containing similar articles on hand in factories and work-shops would much diminish danger from accidents. A common and dangerous practice is hurrying off injured workmen to a hospital in an automobile or other vehicle without giving them any treatment before they leave. Instead of doing this, all large factories and work-shops should have a room set aside furnished with necessary emergency supplies to which injured may be taken and given necessary first-aid treatment. Afterward being attended by a doctor where they are, if their injuries are

so severe that they should not be moved before this is done. Otherwise, being sent home or to a hospital after they have recovered from shock and their injuries have been given proper emergency treatment.

3. INJURIES OF FARM AND RANCH.

While the injuries incident to farm and ranch life are in general terms those which have already been spoken of in the chapter on Common Injuries, a few merit special consideration.

As a means of prevention, it is only necessary to call attention to common care.

Since machinery has come to be more generally used on farms, accidents due to this cause have naturally become more common. They possess no special points of interest in this connection.

The feed-cutter on the farm has always proved dangerous to the hands of the careless. Usually with this the tip of the finger is cleanly cut off. In fact this cut is likely to be so clean that if the finger tip is immediately put in place it not infrequently unites in position so that there is no deformity. This injury should be dressed with a piece of clean gauze and a bandage, and a doctor should be consulted as soon as possible.

An injury not infrequently seen on farms is caused by slipping on a wagon wheel so as to straddle the wheel—thus falling on the crotch. This is a serious injury which demands the attention of a doctor.

Injuries due to goring by wild cattle are not infrequent in handling stock. The horns of these animals often inflict severe wounds with much tearing of the tissues. The abdomen is often torn open. The treatment of wounds of this character has already been described.

Hernia which will be spoken of at length immediately is frequently caused by bucking horses.

Farm and ranch injuries are very commonly made much worse through lack of proper care at the outset. The emergency supplies recommended on page 142 should be found on every farm and ranch.

4. MINING INJURIES.

So large a number of Americans are engaged in mining that a few words on mining injuries will not be out of place here. There is another reason for discussing this subject, however. Largely through the efforts of Dr. M. J. Shields in the Anthracite region of Northeastern Pennsylvania the benefits of first aid have been taught both operators and miners with the happiest results in diminishing the number of unnecessary deaths and in the proper treatment of injuries.

As Doctor Shields teaches, a knowledge of first aid is almost absolutely necessary for miners.

Though certain injuries are of course more frequent in mines, their symptoms and treatment, just as in railway and factory injuries, are exactly like injuries in general.

Causes.

Various: Falls of ore, rock or coal; explosion of gas or powder; being struck by mine cars, or when mules are used kicks from them; electrical shock.

Prevention.

Proper instruction in safety in mining by the company, (Best done by a list of "Don't" printed in various languages and put in the hands of every one employed about a mine.)

Safety appliances provided by the company.

Common care on the part of employed (Remember carelessness on your part may not only result in your own injury, but in that of other people).

General instruction in first aid for employees.

Symptoms.

Are dependent upon the character of the injury.

A miner's injuries are usually produced by the falling of heavy weights and are therefore of a crushing nature. Wounds are torn and are likely to be filled with dirt.

As with railway injuries, on account of the crushing character of mining wounds, hemorrhage is not likely to be severe. Though when the heart begins to recover its strength after the injury, bleeding from torn vessels may be free.

Fractures are common and are not infrequently compound. The bones are likely to be broken in several places. Fracture of the skull is not an uncommon injury. Shock is almost always severe and is the more dangerous as miners frequently must be carried a considerable distance before shock can be treated under favorable conditions.

Burns from explosions of powder or gas are frequent mining injuries.

Treatment.

No new principles are involved.

Shock is always to be remembered and treated.

The emergency supplies required should be as simple as possible as the conditions in mines are such that elaborate equipment can hardly be used. A miner going to render aid to a comrade with two army first-aid packets for wounds, a can of carbolized vaseline for burns and a flask of aromatic spirits of ammonia for shock is well supplied.

At different parts of a mine, boxes of emergency supplies should be found. These should consist of bandages, wooden or wire splints, carbolized vaseline for burns, ½ dozen first-aid packets, a two-ounce bottle of aromatic spirits of ammonia, a graduate and a folding litter. An accident room at a convenient place should also be set aside for every mine where all the emergency supplies named on page 131 should be found.

Severe mining injuries, like other injuries of the same type, require care from a doctor as soon as one can be obtained. Carrying a miner up a narrow shaft presents a peculiar problem in transportation if he must be carried in the upright position. See chapter on Transportation.

5. BUSINESS INJURIES.

Each business has its own peculiar injuries, but only one business injury need be discussed here.

Butchers, or others who cut meat, are very liable to cut their hands and such wounds are likely to prove dangerous. They are commonly infected and are often followed by blood-poisoning. They should be treated like other wounds but should be squeezed so that the blood will wash out the poisonous matter and should never be sealed with collodion or plaster. If severe they demand immediate attention from a doctor, and even if trifling it is safer to consult a physician and if they become inflamed it is exceedingly dangerous not to do so.

HERNIA OR RUPTURE.

This injury is spoken of here because it is usually due to the severe muscular efforts which are incident to hard labor. Naturally, however, such efforts are equally likely to cause hernia wherever they are indulged in.

There is a weak point in the lower part of the abdomen on each side, and occasionally muscular strain, a long breath being taken and the diaphragm fixed, will force a part of the intestines through one of these weak places. Thus a hernia or rupture will be caused. The only method of preventation that can be suggested is the avoidance of such muscular strains, but this of course is hardly practical.

When a hernia occurs there will be a feeling that something has given way and a lump will be found in the groin. As this lump contains intestines it must be handled with the greatest gentleness as rough handling may cause a dangerous injury to the intestines and probably peritonitis.

The patient should be placed on his back with his knees well raised up toward the abdomen and the legs supported with a pillow. Cloths wet in cold water should then be placed over the hernia and a doctor should be sent for as soon as possible.

CHAPTER IX.

INJURIES AND EMERGENCIES OF IN-DOOR AND OUT-DOOR SPORTS.

1. Gymnasium. 2. Baseball. 3. Football. 4. Celebration of July Fourth. 5. Boating, Skating and Swimming. 6. Shooting and Fishing. 7. Automobile. 8. Camping and Summer Outings.

As it is now universally admitted that great physical benefit results to those who engage in healthy sports, the possibility of injuries occurring therein should not be given too heavy weight. The man or boy who enters a physical contest will not go far if he has always before his eyes the possibility of accident. In sport, just as in everything else in life, the successful contestant is he who puts all his energy into making the best possible showing and nothing that is said here should be taken to mean that he should not do this. The risks run are but part of the game and should be accepted as such. Remember that foolhardiness is not courage, however.

There is also one other point which is worthy of consideration here. Violent physical exertion should be gradually prepared for and not rushed into without preparation. A man who is soft has not only soft voluntary muscles, but the muscle of his heart is also soft so that it may be easily strained with perhaps permanent injury. Many of the accidents which we read of as occurring to those engaged in sports are due to their poor physical condition. A man or boy in good training has firm muscles which, to a great extent, prevent his internal organs from blows and falls. Soft muscles cannot do this and with them a trivial blow may prove dangerous.

1. GYMNASIUM.

Bruises, strains, sprains, dislocations and fractures are the commonest gymnasium accidents. The section devoted to these subjects should therefore be studied in connection with them. Boxing is of course responsible for many bruises, especially black eye, which should be treated by the application of cold water or a cold knife-blade. The so-called "alum curd" made by putting powdered alum in milk till a curd is formed is also an excellent application. Both cold and alum contract the vessels and so prevent the escape of more blood. Persons said to be knocked out by blows or falls in gymnasiums will in almost all cases be found to be suffering from shock and should be so treated.

2. BASEBALL.

Severe injuries of the head are sometimes caused by being struck by balls or bats. Blows in the abdomen are also not uncommon. Both should be treated like any other severe injury of the same general character. The services of a doctor should be secured as soon as possible.

Bruises are common but their treatment is not peculiar.

Injuries of the hands and fingers are the commonest baseball injuries. Dislocated and fractured fingers are treated just as are these injuries from other causes.

The name "split finger" is given to the splitting down of the web between the fingers and also to the splitting of the soft tissues of the fingers themselves. Split of the web between the fingers makes generally a clear-cut wound which often bleeds freely. The best way to treat it is to bring the two fingers together and to bandage them in this position without putting anything in contact with the wound itself. This injury should be shown to a doctor.

Splits of the fingers themselves are best dressed with a piece of gauze and a bandage. A surgically clean bandage may be put directly on such a wound. Severe splits of this character should also be shown to a doctor. Shock is sometimes severe in these injuries and should be treated.

The finger-nails are frequently torn partially off by base balls. They should be replaced and held in place by a strip of rubber plaster.

Wounds of the legs and feet, and sometimes of the hands, from the spiked shoes worn by baseball players, are common. So common that it is a serious question if it would not be better to do away with spikes by rule. These spikes make very nasty wounds. After the clothing or shoes and stockings have been removed the part should be immediately covered with gauze and a bandage. Like other wounds, touching such wounds with the hands is likely to prove dangerous.

Shock must often be treated.

These injuries demand attention from a physician.

Emergency supplies are now usually kept at hand by professional and college teams. All that are needed are a few narrow gauze bandages wrapped up so they are kept clean, two first-aid packets, a roll of rubber plaster, a two-ounce bottle of aromatic spirits of ammonia, a sharp knife, a pair of scissors and a few safety and common pins.

3. FOOTBALL.

This, on account of the very severe exertion involved, is the best example of a game which should not be played without careful and gradual preparation.

Bruises, strains, sprains, dislocations and fractures are not particularly uncommon. They are treated exactly like such injuries generally. The knocking out of a football player is usually due either to shock or exhaustion. Men in fine condition recover from slight shock promptly and are again able to take part in the game. Exhaustion always requires rest, and when a man is visibly exhaused it will certainly be better for him, and probably for the eleven, to which he belongs, to take him out of the game.

Of course, at big games doctors are, as they should be, available to treat football injuries.

4. CELEBRATION OF JULY FOURTH.

This celebration is so universally indulged in by young, and sometimes old, America, and the injuries resulting from it are so numerous that it is quite worthy of discussion here. Burning powder, in one way or another, has become such a part of the celebration of July Fourth that it has national sanction, though fortunately for the youth of America some of the more dangerous things which make a noise have been generally prohibited by law.

At the possible risk of appearing unpatriotic it should be stated as my firm belief that more should be done in this direction as the price we still pay annually in injuries and deaths is far too high. This matter can, of course, be regulated to a considerable extent in the individual family and each mother and father should at least see that their children, according to their age, have only fire-crackers or fireworks which they may set off with a reasonable degree of safety. So much has been said in the newspapers of recent years in reference to the dangers of lock-jaw from Fourth-of-July accidents that larger children are not generally deaf to warnings in regard to setting off fire crackers.

Burns, torn wounds from explosions and injuries to the eyes are the commonest Fourth-of-July accidents.

The careful father or mother should not scorn to take the precaution of obtaining a jar of carbolized vaseline and a half-dozen gauze bandages in preparation for the Fourth. Torn wounds demand immediate attention from a doctor on account of possible danger from lock-jaw.

5. BOATING, SKATING AND SWIMMING.

Drowning is the only accident which will be discussed here.

Prevention.

This will be spoken of under two heads: 1. Prevention of accidents that may result in drowning. 2. Rescue of Drowning Persons.

1. **Prevention of Accidents that may result in Drowning.**

Boating accidents are frequent in all parts of the country during the summer season. In order to do your part to prevent them—

Remember: A light boat is not intended for heavy seas; do not change seats except in a wide and steady boat, and above all things do not put yourself in the class of idiots who rock the boat. In case you are thrown into deep water by the turning over of a boat, or from any other cause, do not lose your presence of mind even if you cannot swim. Remember that the water will almost support your weight. Allow yourself to sink low so your nose is just above the water and support yourself by a hand on the boat. Even an oar under the chin will hold you up. If there is nothing which will help to support you, lie flat on the back with the arms stretched out. Especially in salt water with light clothing, one may float almost indefinitely in this position. To do so it is necessary to keep cool if the water or spray rises over the face momentarily. Throwing up the head, or still worse the limbs, to prevent this will result in your sinking.

At the seashore, unless you are a strong swimmer, do not go outside the life-lines and if the undertow is strong be careful that you do not walk out so far that you may be be carried off your feet.

The art of swimming should be made a part of the education of every boy and girl. It is not enough to know how to swim a few strokes. One should at least be able to swim for a few moments while dressed.

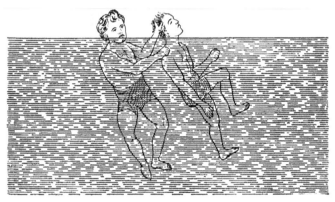

Fig. 35.—1. Rescue of drowning person.

Very cold water and very long swims are likely to result in the exhaustion of even a strong swimmer and are therefore hazardous unless a boat accompanies the swimmer.

2. **Rescue of Drowning Persons.**

If possible, do not attempt to rescue a drowning person in deep water by entering the water yourself. The best interests of the drowning person are served when this is practicable by holding out or throwing something into the water on which he can support himself till he can be pulled ashore or reached in a boat. In case a person has fallen into deep water near the shore take an oar, a pole, a rope or even your coat and hold it out so the drowning person may grasp it. Life preservers, boxes, boards or logs may also be thrown into the water close to the person drowning. As has been stated above, a

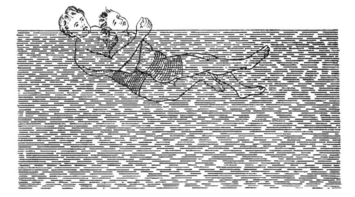

FIG. 36.—2. Rescue of drowning person.

small, floating object is quite sufficient to sustain a person's weight in the water.

If the person in danger of drowning is so far from the shore that the methods just spoken of cannot be used you must enter the water to rescue him. Take off as much of your clothing as possible. It is especially necessary to rid yourself of your shoes. If you are not a strong swimmer it will be much better to support yourself with a life preserver, a board, box, or the like when

swimming out to the drowning person.   Always take care
not to permit him to grasp you, for this may result in
drowning you both.   If he succeeds in seizing you it
will be safest to allow yourself to sink or to strike him a
blow in the face in order to make him loosen his hold.
There is no cruelty in such a blow; it may be his only
salvation.   Unconscious persons are in fact rescued
much more easily.

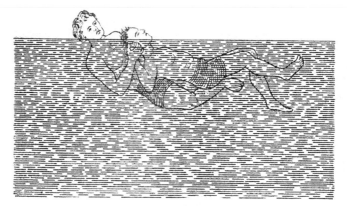

Fig. 37.--3. Rescue of drowning person.

Always approach a drowning man from behind, grasp his
hair or collar with your left hand and his right shoulder
with your right hand keeping him at arm's length with his
mouth and nose just above the water, then "tread water."
As soon as you can, seize his right wrist and pull it behind
his head, then take a few strokes to get on your back,
at the same time pull the person you are rescuing on your
chest and start to swim backward to shore.   Swim as low

as possible, with your face and that of the drowning person, just out of the water.

To rescue a person who has broken through the ice: You should first tie a rope around your body and have the other end tied, or held, on shore. Then secure a long board, or a ladder, crawl out on this or push it out so that the person in the water may reach it. If nothing can be found on which you can support your weight do not at-

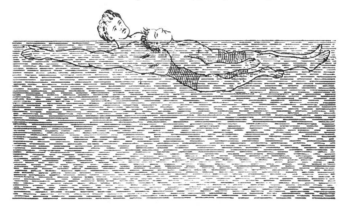

Fig. 38.—4. Rescue of drowning person.

tempt to walk out toward the person to be rescued, but lie down flat on your face and crawl out as by doing this much less weight bears at any one point on the ice than in walking.

Symptoms.

Are of course those of suffocation. In addition a frothy fluid is often noticed in the mouth and nose and the body is cold.

Treatment.

Is naturally that of suffocation in general preceded by that necessary to get rid of the water which has entered the windpipe and lungs. Also afterward necessary measures to restore warmth to the body.

In order that the proper treatment for drowning may be given promptly, the necessary directions should be posted at all boat-houses and bath-houses.

As soon as the nearly drowned person has been taken from the water loosen all tight clothing, at the same time send some one else for a doctor and for dry clothing and blankets when possible. Quickly clean mud or water from the mouth with a handkerchief on the finger.

Turn the patient on his face, clasp your hands around his waist, raise him up by the middle and keep him elevated for a few seconds in order to allow water to drain out of throat and lungs.

Turn patient flat on his back.

Pull out tongue by grasping it with a dry cloth. Have some one else hold it out. Or if alone, if possible, tie in this position with a bandage or rubber band over the tongue and under the jaw. The reason for pulling the tongue forward is because in an unconscious person it is likely to fall back and block the windpipe.

Perform artificial respiration. The Sylvester method is best.

First put a pad, such as a rolled up coat, under the shoulders. This helps to expand the chest. Do not allow the head to hang back so as to strain the windpipe; if necessary, a little pad under the head may be used to prevent this. Kneel just above patient's head, catch both his arms just below the elbows. Draw the arms

outward and upward gently and steadily and hold them
as far as they will go above head for about 2 seconds.

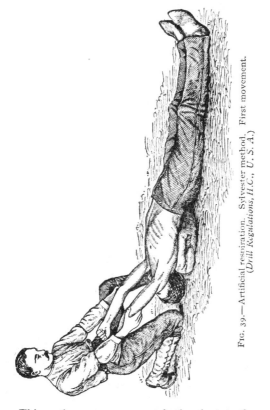

FIG. 39.—Artificial respiration. Sylvester method. First movement.
(*Drill Regulations, H.C., U. S. A.*)

This motion opens or expands the chest to the greatest
possible extent.

This is due to the fact that certain muscles are attached to both arms and ribs and when the arms are raised these muscles raise the ribs and so enlarge the chest.

Then bring the arms down till the elbows press against the chest, a little pressure will diminish the size of the elastic chest as much as possible. Do this for about 2 seconds.

Continue these motions about fifteen times per minute. Keep this up till the patient begins to breath himself. Persons have been restored after several hours of artificial respiration and after they have been in the water for some time.

Artificial Respiration when done properly is hard work for the operator and he should be relieved by someone else as soon as he grows tired.

A valuable addition to this method of artificial respiration is the Laborde Method, which consists of Rhythmic Traction of the Tongue. Another person is required for this. He seizes the tongue and draws it out as far as he can each time that the arms are extended over the head, and allows it to recede into the mouth as the arms go down, keeping this up as long as artificial respiration is continued.

At the same time that one or two persons are performing artificial respiration, without interfering with them, others should remove the patient's wet clothing and dry him with towels or something else, then covering him with a dry coat or blanket.

As soon as the patient begins to breathe himself, but not before, his limbs should be well rubbed toward the heart under the blankets. This will help to restore the circulation.

He should afterward be put to bed well covered and surrounded with hot bottles. The windows should be opened

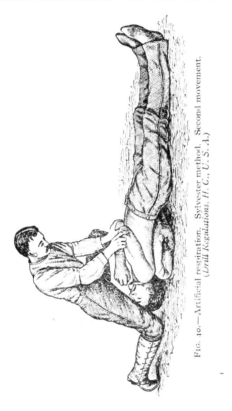

FIG. 40.—Artificial respiration. Sylvester method. Second movement. (*Drill Regulations, H. C., U. S. A.*)

so that he may have plenty of air. When he can swallow, hot stimulants should be given him.

After the danger is over the patient should be allowed to sleep quietly.

Warning.

If the breathing stops at any time after it has once begun you must immediately start again with artificial respiration.

6. SHOOTING AND FISHING.

Shooting accidents are common and generally result from carelessness in the use of rifles or shot-guns.

Shooting.

Prevention.

Never put a cartridge or shell into the chamber before you need it and always remove it when the need for it ceases.

Do not cock a gun except when you expect to shoot at any moment and uncock it when this necessity ceases. Never point a gun, whether loaded or unloaded, toward yourself or anyone else. Be particularly careful in going over or through fences, and in boats.

When hunting in company try to know where your companions are at all times and do not fire in that direction. Make sure in firing at anything in the woods that your are not shooting at a man.

Symptoms.

Wounds from rifles have already been described as punctured wounds. Wounds from shot-guns received near the muzzle are tearing wounds with great destruction of the tissues and often actually tear off parts of the body. At a far distance shot may lodge just under the skin or may only produce a bruise with a stinging sensation.

Treatment.

For the trivial injuries which have just been mentioned the services of a doctor are never immediately necessary, though when shot has lodged under the skin, a doctor should always remove it, as blood-poisoning may follow attempts to do so by other persons.

With serious shot-gun or rifle injuries circumstances are usually such that a doctor cannot be obtained promptly, though one should be secured as soon as possible. A comrade of the injured man will, therefore, almost always be compelled to give necessary treatment. This does not differ in any respect from the treatment of such wounds due to other causes. The bleeding may be very severe, however and must be checked at any cost, even if the wound will probably be infected in doing so.

Shock always demands treatment.

Fishing.

A fishhook caught in the flesh, if the barb is not engaged, is easily removed. If the barb is firmly fixed, however, quite the contrary is true. In this case the point of the hook should be pushed through till the barb has passed through and out of the skin. The barb should then be cut off with a strong pair of nippers. Such a wound should, when possible, be shown to a doctor, as it is very likely to become inflamed. If this occurs a doctor's services are always required. In any event, the wound should be put in hot water, which, if possible, has been previously boiled, and squeezed so as to squeeze out poisonous matter. Such a wound should never be sealed with collodion or plaster, but should be dressed with a surgically clean or antiseptic compress or bandage.

7. AUTOMOBILE.

Automobile injuries are becoming increasingly common on account of the more general use of the automobile.

Such injuries are usually bruises, strains, sprains, dislocations, fractures or wounds, and are likely to be very severe and of a crushing or mangling character

Prevention.

Every owner of a car should himself know or have some responsible person in his employ who is able to recognize whether his automobile is in fit condition to run with safety. Automobile accidents due to the most obvious defects in the mechanism of machines are far too common.

High speed, especially at night and on poor roads, is responsible for many accidents. Slippery roads demand especial care on the part of the driver, on account of the danger from skidding.

The use of alcoholic liquors by drivers of automobiles is as much, if not more, dangerous than similar indulgence on the part of locomotive engineers.

Grade crossings of railways should be approached by the automobilist with the greatest care, as accidents due to collisions with railway trains are very common.

The **Symptoms** and **Treatment** of automobile injuries need not be described as they are exactly the same as with similar injuries due to other causes.

8. CAMPING AND SUMMER OUTINGS.

A number of not closely related injuries and emergencies will be discussed under this heading. None are peculiar either to life in camp or to summer outings, but do occur more commonly under such conditions. As out-of-door active life is also not infrequently accompanied by injuries, such as bruises, strains, sprains, dislocations, fractures and wounds, these should also be studied in this connection.

This section comprises: Sunburn, Mosquito bites, Stings of Insects, Poison Ivy, Plant poisons, especially Mushrooms, Bites of Snakes, Injuries of feet, Cramps in legs.

Sunburn.

This may vary from a slight redness of the skin to a very severe burn. Persons with delicate skins may avoid a good deal of needless discomfort and pain by protecting themselves when exposed to the bright summer sun. That there is anything healthy in sunburn or tan is a wholly false idea. The measures of protection are naturally the use of hats and clothing which shade the face and body from the sun. Wetting the face, especially with salt water, is likely to cause very severe sunburn. Any toilet powder will protect the face from the sun's rays to some extent. though the pink Calamid powder is undoubtedly the best.

The treatment consists of soothing applications; ordinary or carbolized vaselin may be used. An excellent application and one easily prepared is 1 part lime-water to 3 parts almond or olive oil.

Mosquito Bites.

These injuries are usually regarded as of trivial importance, but it is well to remember in malarial districts that malaria is caused by mosquitoes and that to prevent this disease mosquito nets and other means of protection against them should be used.

Ammonia is the best remedy, as the poison is an acid one. Lime-water with two drops of carbolic acid to the ounce is also good. Menthol and toilet powder often give temporary relief.

Stings and Bites of Insects and Spiders.

These are rarely dangerous to life, though they may cause a great deal of pain and discomfort. Nothing need be said in reference to prevention or symptoms. Ammonia should be immediately applied to the part where the sting entered; this should be removed if it remains in the wound. Afterward cool, wet dressings should be used. Cloths wet with water in which a very few drops of carbolic acid have been thoroughly mixed, wet salt and wet earth are all good applications.

Poison Ivy or Oak.

These plants which so commonly cause skin poisoning belong to the sumac family. Two varieties are described—one, a shrub or small tree, with oval, pointed leaves arranged in clusters of from seven to thirteen on a common stalk; the other is a creeper or a climbing plant with broad leaves, sometimes slightly notched, arranged in clusters of three. Both have berries.

These plants cause poisoning in almost every one if touched, and some persons can scarcely go near them without being poisoned. Early in an attack a person may convey the disease from one part of his body to another, and extremely rarely one person infects another.

Prevention.

Is naturally avoiding poison ivy or oak. Remember there is no certainty that if you have handled these plants at one time without injury that the same will be true on another occasion.

Symptoms.

Are those of a severe inflammation of the skin. This, of course, appears more often on the exposed parts, usually the hands and arms and the face. The skin becomes much inflamed and swollen, blisters form and even pus sometimes. There may be loss of the upper layers of the skin and a red, weepy surface. The pain, itching and discomfort are severe. The symptoms, as a whole, are very violent.

Treatment.

If severe, a doctor should be consulted promptly. A very good and simple treatment is a wash of a two or three per cent. boracic acid solution followed by the ordinary zinc ointment. Lime-water for the wash and carbolized vaselin for the ointment are fairly good remedies. The ointment should be washed off daily with the wash, the part dried gently and the ointment reapplied.

Plant Poisons, Especially Mushrooms.

A number of the common plants are poisonous. Among them are Bitter Sweet, Deadly Night Shade, Mountain Ash, Hemlock, Hellebore, Jamestown Weed, Wild Parsley and Lettuce and certain Mushrooms and Toadstools. Cases of poisoning, except from the last, are rare.

A rule which should always be observed is never to eat anything growing unless you are very sure that you know that it is not poisonous and to prevent children from doing so.

Mushroom, sometimes called toadstool poisoning, is commonly due to faliure to distinguish between the poisonous and non-poisonous varieties.

The rules which are commonly accepted for doing so are as follows:

Consider dangerous all mushrooms which have:

1. "A cup-like formation at the base of stem (so-called death cup)."

2. "A scaly or close-fitting layer at the base of the stem.

3. "Loose warts on the cap."

4. "A milky juice (unless this is red.)"

5. "Great brittleness, with gills nearly all of equal length and the flesh of the cap thin."

6. "A honeycombed appearance of the gills, if the flesh tastes bitter, or the mouths of the tubes are reddish, or the flesh changes color when cut or bruised."

7. "A cobwebby veil or ring when the plant is young."

8. "A slimy cap and clay-colored spores" (Dulles).

Moreover, all mushrooms that are decaying or are in the immature button stage should be discarded.

Symptoms of Poisoning from Growing Plants.

Nausea and vomiting. Severe pain in abdomen. Great depression. Unconsciousness, sometimes weak pulse, shallow respiration.

Delirium from some poisons.

Treatment.

Send for doctor.

Cause vomiting.

Stimulants.

Rest in lying-down position, with head low.

Cover warmly and apply heat by means of hot bottles around patient.

Snake Bite.

Snake bites are exceedingly rare injuries in this country, but bites from poisonous snakes are so rapidly fatal if not promptly given proper attention that it is necessary for the student of first aid to know how to treat them. The rattlesnake and the moccasin are probably most generally to be feared in the United States. Neither is equally virulent at all seasons of the year.

Prevention.

When it is impossible to avoid the localities where poisonous snakes are commonly found, comprises the wearing of high boots or leggings by day and sleeping on a cot or raised platform at night instead of on the ground. The Mexican plan when sleeping on the ground of surrounding the sleeper with a hair rope or lariat is undoubtedly a good one, as snakes will not cross such a rope.

Symptoms.

Great pain in wound. Rapid swelling. Much depression and weakness, followed promptly by death in some cases unless proper treatment is given.

Treatment.

Immediately to tie a string, handkerchief or bandage between the bitten part and the body if this is practicable. Naturally, this can only be done in the extremities. This cutting off of the return of the blood to the body, of course, prevents absorption of the poison. The wound should then be soaked in hot water if this is obtainable and in any event squeezed, milked or sucked. This is for the purpose of extracting as much poison as possible. Sucking the wound is not dangerous unless one has cuts or scrapes in the mouth. These proceedures should not be delayed for a moment in order to send for a doctor but one should be summoned as soon as possible. The further first-aid treatment consists of cauterizing or burning the wound with ammonia. Strong ammonia should be used for this purpose if it can be procured. The patient should also be dosed with stimulants. It is not necessary to give whisky or brandy so as to intoxicate him. But a large drink of whisky or brandy or a full dose of aromatic spirits of ammonia should be given at once and should be repeated as often as seems necessary to keep up the strength of the patient. Do not be afraid to give too much for persons bitten by poisonous snakes require a large amount of stimulants.

Leave the string or bandage tied above the wound in place as long as you dare. After an hour, however, if no doctor has arrived you must remember that your tight bandage is likely to cause mortification as it has cut off the circulation. Do not try to remove it at once, loosen it a trifle so that a little poison escapes to the body then tighten it again and repeat after a few moments. If the patient does not seem to be greatly affected by the poison you will finally be able to remove the constricting band entirely. But, on the other hand, if the poison which escapes into the body seriously depresses the patient you must keep the bitten part tied off and take the chance of mortification.

Injuries of the Feet and Cramps in the Legs.

The pleasures of a camping trip which requires much walking depends to a great extent on the condition of the feet.

The importance of well-fitting shoes cannot be overestimated. The shoes should have heavy soles, moderate heels and be neither tight nor loose though they should be tightly laced and longer than the feet. New and stiff shoes are almost sure to be very uncomfortable; shoes should be worn sufficiently beforehand so that they will have adapted themselves to the shape of the feet. Cotton is the best material for the socks or stockings and they must be long enough so that the toes have free play. Great care should be taken to have any darns smooth. The feet should be carefully washed and dried after a day's walk and clean socks or stockings should be put on. If the feet are swollen or hot, wash them with warm salt water or alcohol before putting on fresh hose. Talcum powder will prevent foot troubles. In the morning dry the feet thoroughly, rub on the powder and shake a good amount in each shoe.

Blisters are best treated by washing the foot thoroughly in hot water, then taking a clean needle and pricking the blister, not directly, but through the skin at the side, and gently pressing out the fluid in the blister till it is flat.

To toughen and harden the feet soak them for some time in a bowl of cold tannic acid solution, a tablespoonful of the acid to a bowl of water. A solution of alcohol and salt answers the same purpose.

Cramps in the leg-muscles often come on after unusual exertion. They are best treated by rubbing and kneading the muscles. Wrapping the legs in hot cloths will also assist.

The emergency supplies for a camp should, if possible, be those already given for the household. They may, however, be somewhat cut down in bulk and number in case of necessity. The minimum should be:

Aromatic Spirits of Ammonia, 2 oz. bottle, rubber cork.
Syrup of Ginger, 2 oz.
Seidlitz Powders, 12 in tin box.
5 gr. Bismuth Subnitrate tablets (200).
$\frac{1}{10}$ gr. Calomel tablets (50).
Carbolized Vaseline, 1 tin.
Oil of Cloves, 1 Drachm bottle, labelled "Poison."
Soda Mint tablets, 50.
1 Tin Talcum Powder.
1 Small package Antiseptic Gauze.
2 U. S. Army First-aid Dressings.
1 box Tooth wax.
1 box Tooth plaster.

12

1 box Corn plaster.
1 Sharp knife.
1 Pair scissors.
Needles and pins, ordinary and safety.
Thread.

CHAPTER X.

TRANSPORTATION OF WOUNDED, INJURED AND SICK.

A man trained in first aid will usually find when he has treated a wound or injury or has cared for a sick person that his duty is but half performed. Accidents and emergency cases of sickness usually occur in places from which it is absolutely necessary to carry patients, and even in his home the patient must frequently be transferred to his bed. Unless the proper means for transporting patients are understood and practiced very grave harm may result to them. In fact, the benefits from good first-aid treatment may be undone by bad transportation.

It should be understood of course that whatever method of transportation is adopted, first aid should be given before it is attempted, and that when necessary the clothing should be loosened so that it will not constrict the neck, chest nor abdomen during transportation.

The kind of transportation which should be furnished must of course vary widely with the character of the complaint. All serious cases of illness or injury should be carried on litters whenever it is possible to procure or to improvise them and in case of doubt it is always much safer when practicable to carry the patient lying down.

The ordinary type of litter is so well known that it hardly need be described. It consists of two long poles with a bed usually made of canvas between them and cross-pieces to keep the long poles apart and thus to stretch the canvas. The poles are long enough to afford handholds for the bearers at each end of the litter.   Fairly satisfactory litters may be improvised.   The easiest one of these to make usually is the coat litter.   For this two coats and a pair of poles are needed.   The sleeves of the coats are first turned inside out and the coats are then placed on the ground with their lower edges touching each other, the poles are passed through the sleeves on each side, the coats are buttoned up and the buttoned side turned down.   Two poles and a large blanket or rug may also be used to make a litter.   The blanket or rug is spread on the ground with the two poles at the edges of its long sides.   These edges are then rolled on the poles till a distance of about 20 inches is left between them.   This litter may be turned over before being used, and especially with narrow blankets or rugs it is much safer to bind them to the poles with twine.   With both these litters it is desirable, when possible, to tie on two pieces of wood for cross-pieces so as to prevent the poles from approaching each other when the weight of the patient is put on the litter.

Instead of rugs and blankets, bags and sacks may be employed for litter beds.   The bottoms of the latter should be ripped so that the poles may be passed through the number sufficient to give the length of litter required.

With these and similar litters careful tests should be made before allowing them to be used for patients; care is also necessary to guard against accidents during transportation.   Numbers of articles, some of which may almost always be easily procured, may also be used for litters in case of necessity.   Such articles are doors, window shutters, boards, bed frames, benches, ladders, mattresses, rugs, blankets and mats.

Whatever the type of litter, used the greatest gentleness should be observed in transferring the patient to it, and unless he is to be subjected to unnecessary suffering all his bearers must work in unison.   The necessity for bearers working together has been so thoroughly appreciated by all the armies of the world that they all now give a regular litter drill to men charged with the duty of carrying wounded. It would hardly be possible to improve on the United States Army Drill Regulations on this subject which will therefore be quoted at length. Slight changes in arrangement have been made as well as a few omissions. The effort required to learn this drill will well repay anyone who really desires to be proficient in first-aid work.

In the army each litter squad consists of two men. No. 1 is at the right when in line, and No. 2 at the left. In carrying the litter No. 1 marches in front, and No. 2 in rear.

It is now understood that the litter has been opened and placed near the patient.

THE LOADED LITTER.
To load and unload the Litter.

1. The litter being at the *open*, the patient, with two bearers, must always be carried to it. This may be done in either of two ways.

2. The litter being at the *open*, the instructor or No. 2 commands:

1. Right (Left) side, 2. Posts.

If the command is *right side, posts*, the bearers go to right side of patient and take positions, No. 1 at the right thigh and No. 2 at the right shoulder, facing the patient. If the command is *left*, they take similar positions on the left side.

3.   1. Prepare to lift, 2. Lift.

At the first command the bearers kneel on the knee nearest the patient's feet. No. 1 passes one arm under the hips and the other beneath the knees; No. 2 passes one hand under the patient's

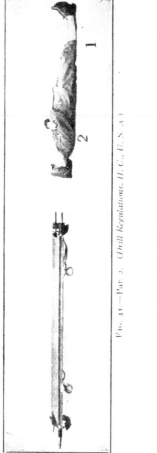

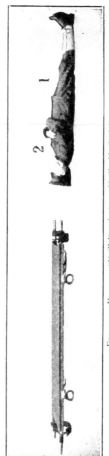

Fig. 41.—Par. 2. (Drill Regulations, H. C., U. S. A.)

Fig. 42.—Par. 2. (Drill Regulations, H. C., U. S. A.)

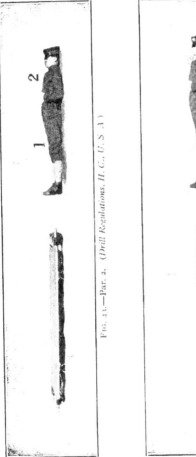

Fig. 43.—Par. 2. (Drill Regulations, H. C., U. S. A.)

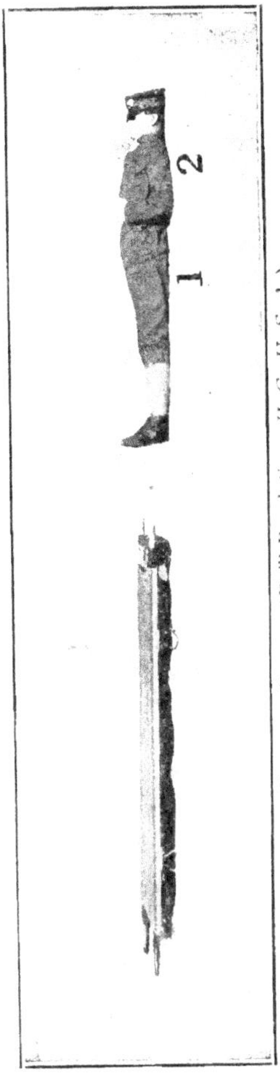

Fig. 44.—Par. 2. (Drill Regulations, H. C., U. S. A.)

shoulders to the further armpit, and the other arm beneath the small of the back.

At *lift*, they lift together, slowly and carefully, raising the patient upon their knees, then readjusting their hold, rise to their feet and carry the patient by the shortest route to the side of the litter, when the squad is *halted*.

4.   1. *Lower*, 2. **Patient.**

At *patient*, the bearers kneel and place the patient on their knees; they stoop forward and lower him gently upon the litter; they then

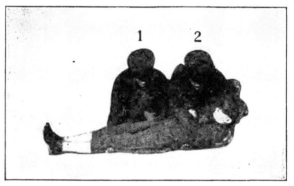

FIG. 45.—Par. 3.   (*Drill Regulations, H. C., U. S. A.*)

rise, and at once resume their positions at *litter posts*, without command.

(Litter Posts: Nos. 1 and 2 take posts between the front and rear handles, respectively, facing the front. The foot or front of a loaded litter is always the end corresponding to the feet of the patient.)

Should it be necessary in emergencies to use three bearers, this may be done with similar commands, by having the third bearer placed at the patient in such a way that he may support the knees and legs.

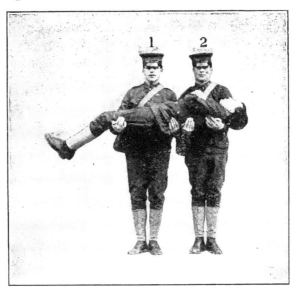

FIG. 46.—Par. 3.   (*Drill Regulations, H. C., U. S. A.*)

5.   1. *Hips*, 2. **Posts.**

At *posts*, No. 1 proceeds to the patient's right hip and No. 2 to the left hip, facing the patient.

6.   1. *Prepare to lift*, 2. **Lift.**

At the first command, the bearers kneel on the knee nearest the patient's feet, they then raise him to a sitting position, and pass each one hand and arm around his back, while the other hands are passed under the thighs, grasping each other. The patient, if able, clasps his arms around the bearers' necks. At *lift*, they lift the patient, both rising together, and carry him to the centre of the side of the litter where the squad is halted.

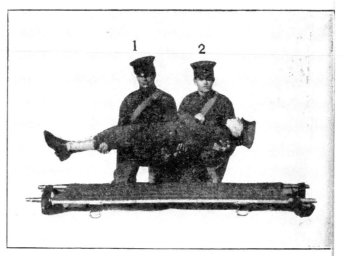

FIG. 47.—Par. 4. (*Drill Regulations, H. C., U. S. A.*)

7.   1. *Lower*, 2. **Patient**.

At *patient*, the bearers stoop and lower the patient upon the litter to a sitting position, the patient releasing his hold around the bearers' necks. No. 2 then passes his left hand across the front of the patient's chest to the opposite armpit and grasps the patient. No. 1 releases his hold at the right side of patient, steps astride of patient's lower extremities and grasps the patient's right and left thighs just above the knee with his left and right hands, respectively. Both bearers then turn and lower the patient upon the litter, head toward No. 2, and take their positions at *litter posts* without command.

8. To *unload* posts are taken and the patient lifted in the same way and by the same commands. At *hips posts* the bearers take

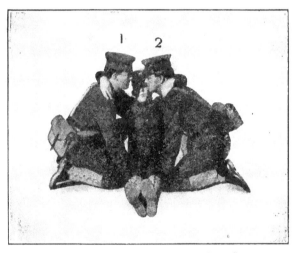

Fig. 48.—Par. 6. (*Drill Regulations, H. C., U. S. A.*)

their posts at the sides of the litter and at *prepare to lift* they lift the patient to a sitting position on the side of the litter by reversing the movements heretofore described and then take the position of prepare to lift.

The bearers move backward if at *side posts* and forward if at *hip posts*, until clear of the litter, when they *halt* and *lower patient*.

POSITION OF PATIENT ON THE LITTER.

9. The position of a patient on the litter depends on the character of his injury. An overcoat, blanket, or other suitable and convenient article should be used as a pillow to give support and slightly raised position to the head. If the patient is faint the head should be kept low. Difficulty of breathing in wounds of the chest

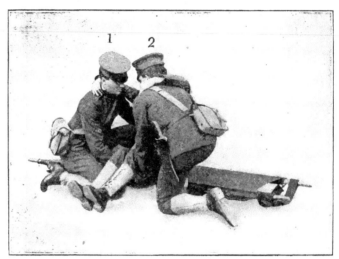

Fig. 49.—Par. 7. (*Drill Regulations, H. C., U. S. A.*)

is relieved by a sufficient padding underneath. In wounds of the abdomen the best position is on the injured side, or on the back if the front of the abdomen is injured, the legs in either case being drawn up, and a pillow or other available object placed under the knees to keep them bent.

In an injury of the upper extremity calling for litter transportation, the best position is on the back with the injured arm laid over the body or suitably placed by its side, or on the uninjured side with the wounded arm laid over the body. In injuries of the lower extremity the patient should be on his back, or inclining toward the wounded side; in case of fracture of either lower extremity, if a splint cannot be applied, it is always well to bind both limbs together.

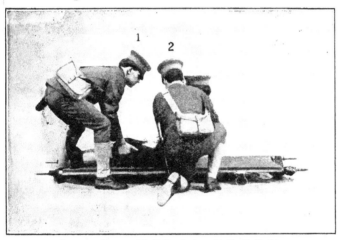

FIG. 50.—Par. 7. (*Drill Regulations, H. C., U. S. A.*)

GENERAL DIRECTIONS.

10. In moving the patient either with or without the litter, every movement should be made deliberately and as gently as possible, having special care not to jar the injured part. The command *steady* will be used to prevent undue haste or other irregular movements.

11. *The loaded litter should never be lifted or lowered without orders.*

MOVEMENTS OF THE LOADED LITTER ARE EXECUTED AS FOLLOWS:

12.   1. *Prepare to Lift,* 2. **Lift.**

At the first command the bearers without facing about (they are in the position of Litter Posts) stoop and firmly grasp the handles of the litter; at lift they slowly rise erect.

13.   *At the Command,* 1. **Forward,** 2. **March.**

The bearers step off, No. 1 with the left and No. 2 with the right foot, taking short sliding steps of about 20 inches, to avoid jolting and to secure a uniform motion to the litter.

14.   *Being at the Lift,* 1. **Lower,** 2. **Litter.**

At litter the bearers lower the litter to the ground. The litter should be lifted and lowered slowly and without jerk, both ends simultaneously, the rear bearer moving in accord with the front bearer, so as to maintain the canvas horizontal.

15. The rear bearer should watch the movements of the front bearer and time his own by them, so as to insure ease and steadiness of action.

16. The number of steps per minute will depend on the weight carried and other conditions affecting each individual case.

17. The handles of the litter should be held in the hands at arm's length. Only under most exceptional conditions should the handles be supported on the shoulders.

18. The bearers should keep the litter level notwithstanding any unevenness of the ground.

19. As a rule, the patient should be carried on the litter feet foremost, but in going up hill his head should be in front. In case of fracture of the lower extremities, he is carried uphill feet foremost and downhill head foremost to prevent the weight of the body from pressing down on the injured part.

To Pass Obstacles.

20. A breach should be made in a fence or wall for the passage of the litter. If there is no gate or other opening, or should it be necessary to surmount the obstacle, the latter being not over 3 feet high, the litter is *halted* and *lowered*, when the commands are given:

1. *At sides of litter*, 2. **Posts.**

At *posts*, Nos. 1 and 2 take posts on the right and left of the litter, respectively, at the center and facing it.

21.   1. *Prepare to lift*, 2. **Lift**, 3. **March.**

At the first command the bearers stoop and seize their respective poles with both hands; at *lift*, the litter is lifted, and at *march*, it is advanced to the obstacle and passed over until the front stirrups have cleared it. The litter is there rested, while No. 2 steps around between the rear handles which he supports, No. 1 getting over the obstacle; No. 1 takes the front handles facing the litter and together the bearers pass the litter over until the rear handles rest on the obstacle, when No. 2 gets over, taking left front handle, and both resuming *at sides of litter posts*, move the litter forward until free of the obstacle, when they *halt* and *lower litter*, and resume *litter posts* without command.

22. The passage of a cut or ditch not over 3 feet deep is effected in a similar manner, but without special command. The litter being *halted* and *lowered* at its edge, No. 1 descends into the ditch and takes hold of the front handles, facing the litter. Both bearers then support and advance the litter until only the rear stirrups or handles rest upon the edge, when No. 2 descends and the litter is carried across. *These directions are general.*

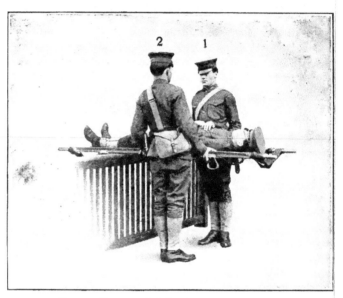

FIG. 51.—Par. 21.   (*Drill Regulations, H. C., U. S. A.*)

BEARER WORK WITH INCREASED NUMBERS.*

23. Under exceptional circumstances, as in ascending or descending stairs, when the patient is very heavy, the ground difficult, or an obstacle over 3 feet high has to be surmounted, it may be necessary to use additional bearers.

24. When three bearers are available, the third bearer gives aid where most needed; in loading and unloading he usually places the litter under the patient or removes it, but he may assist in

*The positions of the numbers of the additional squads are shown in the plates by Roman numerals.

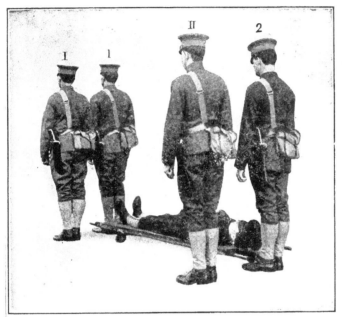

FIG. 52.—Par. 25. (*Drill Regulations, H. C., U. S. A.*)

supporting a fractured limb. In litter bearing he acts as a relay or assists in supporting either end of the litter as directed.

25. When necessary to use an additional squad, the first squad being at *litter posts*, the commands are given:

1. *Additional squad*, 2. *Litter*, 3. **Posts.**

The post of the additional squad is on the left of the litter close to it and facing the front. No. 1 by the front handle and No. 2 by the rear handle; No. 2 of the first squad is in command.

13

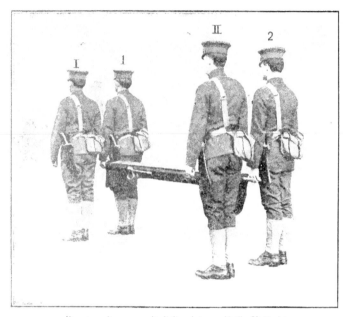

FIG. 54.—Par. 28. (Drill Regulations, H. C., U. S. A.)

26. To change posts, the litter being at the *lower:*

1. *Change.* 2. **Posts.**

At *posts,* the squads change places, retaining their relative positions in the squad.

27. To change bearers, litter at the *carry:*

1. *Change,* 2. **Bearers.**

At *bearers,* the litter is shifted from one squad to the other, the position of the squads remaining unchanged.

28. To carry the litter by four bearers, the litter being *lowered* and the squads at *litter posts:*

1. *Four bearers*, 2. *Litter*, 3. **Posts.**

At *posts*, the first squad steps outside the right handles of the litter, facing the front and opposite the additional squad.

29. 1. *Prepare to lift*, 2. **Lift.**

At the first command all stoop and grasp with one hand the handle nearest them and at *lift* rise erect.

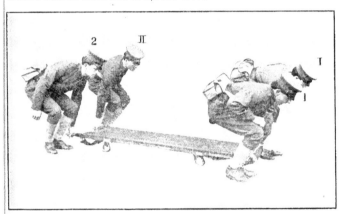

FIG. 54.—Par. 29. (*Drill Regulations, H. C., U. S. A.*)

30. To surmount an obstacle over 3 feet high, the litter being lifted by *four bearers* (two squads) the commands are given:

1. *Raise*, 2. **Litter**, 3. **March.**

At the second command the bearers face the litter, grasp the handles with both hands, and carefully raise it to the level of the obstacle; at *march* they carry it over until the front stirrups have cleared, where it is rested.   The front bearers cross the obstacle and resume hold of the handles on the other side; the litter is then

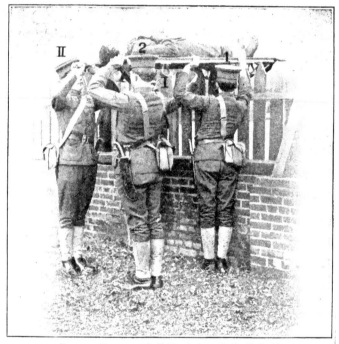

FIG. 55.—Par. 30.   (*Drill Regulations, H. C., U. S. A.*)

advanced until only the rear handles rest on the obstacle, when the rear bearers get over and resume hold of their handles; the litter is then *halted* and *lowered*.

31.   When it is necessary to use four bearers to load, the commands are:

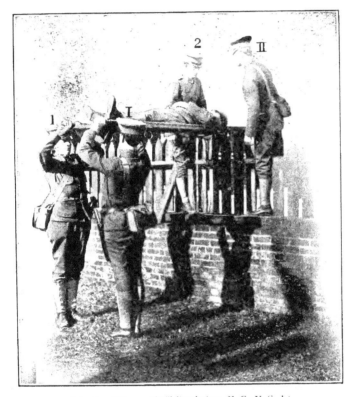

FIG. 56.—Par. 30. (*Drill Regulations, H. C., U. S. A.*)

1. *Four bearers.* 2. *Right (left) side.* 3. **Posts.**

At *posts;* the first squad take their usual posts (par. 2); No. 1 of the additional squad takes post opposite No. 1 of the first squad, and No. 2 at the right (left) ankle.

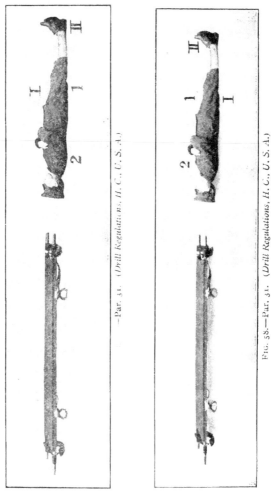

FIG. 58.—Par. 31. (Drill Regulations, H. C., U. S. A.)

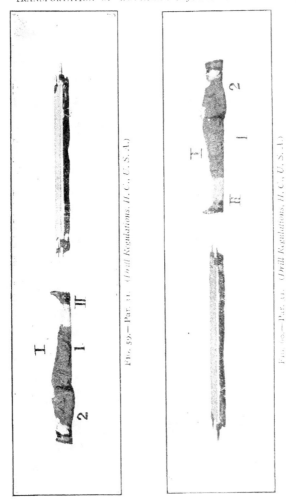

Fig. 59.— Par. 31. (Drill Regulations, H. C., U. S. A.)

Fig. 60.— Par. 31. (Drill Regulations, H. C., U. S. A.)

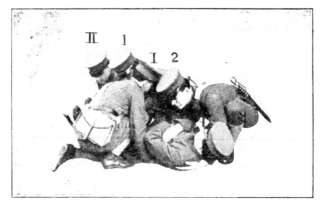

FIG. 61.—Par. 32.   (*Drill Regulations, H. C., U. S. A.*)

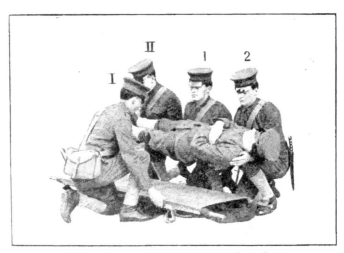

FIG. 62.—Par. 32.   (*Drill Regulations, H. C., U. S. A.*)

32.   1. *Prepare to lift,* 2. **Lift.**

At the first command all the bearers kneel on the knee nearest the patient's feet (right knee if on the right of the patient, and on the left knee if on his left); No. 2, second squad, passes both forearms under the patient's legs, carefully supporting the fracture, if there be one; the Nos. 1 pass their arms under the small of his back and thighs, not locking hands; No. 2, first squad, passes one hand under his neck to the farther armpit, with the other supporting the nearer shoulder.

At the second command all lift together slowly and carefully and place the patient upon the knees of the three bearers. As soon as he is firmly supported there, the bearer on the free side relinquishes his hold, passes quickly and by the shortest line to the litter, which he takes up by the middle, one pole in each hand, and returning rapidly, places it under the patient and against the bearers' ankles.

33.   1. *Lower,* 2. **Patient.**

The free bearer stoops and assists the other numbers in gently and carefully lowering the patient upon the litter. The bearers the rise and at once resume their positions at *litter posts* (par. 28).

34. To unload, posts are taken at patient as in loading. At the commands:

1. *Prepare to lift,* 2. **Lift,**

the patient is lifted and placed upon the knees of the three bearers, as in par. 32, the free bearer then removes the litter, and at *lower patient* all lower him carefully to the ground.

To Carry a Loaded Litter Upstairs.

35. The loaded litter is usually carried upstairs head first, and downstairs, feet first.

To carry loaded litter upstairs: Two squads are required for this movement. The litter is marched to the foot of the stairs in the usual manner, *wheeled about, halted*, and *lowered*.   It is then lifted by four bearers (par. 28–29), using both hands when necessary, and carried up.   The litter must be kept as level as possible,

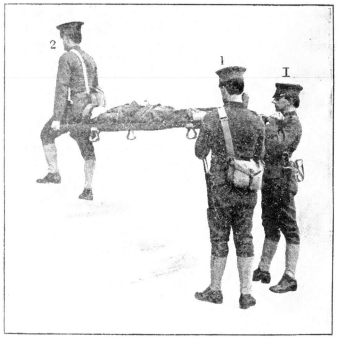

FIG. 63.—Par. 37.   (*Drill Regulations, H. C., U. S. A.*)

the upper bearers lowering and the lower bearers raising their ends for this purpose and being careful to see that the litter is not tilted.

To Carry a Loaded Litter Downstairs.

36. The litter is carried downstairs in the same manner as it is carried upstairs, except that it is not wheeled about.

37. When for any reason it is necessary to use three bearers, the commands 1. *Three bearers, prepare to lift*, 2. **Lift,** are used. At the first command the additional bearer takes post outside the

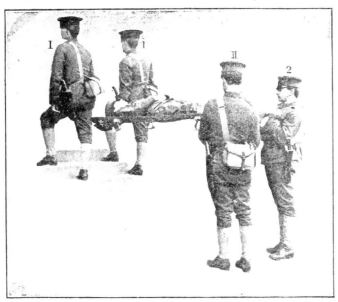

Fig. 64.—Par. 35.   (*Drill Regulations, H. C., U. S. A.*)

left handle at the foot of the litter, opposite No. 1, who steps outside the right handle. Both face the litter, stoop, and grasp their respective poles. No. 2 faces about, stoops, and grasps his handles. At *lift*, the litter is lifted and carried up (or down) the stairs.   If the litter is to be carried downstairs by three bearers, No. 2 does not face about.

FROM LITTER TO BED.

38. The litter is placed at the foot of the bed, as nearly as possible in line with it, and the patient is transferred to the bed, as described in par. 8.   Often it is simpler, after the patient is lifted, to roll the bed in front of the bearers, who then lower the patient upon it.   If there is no fracture or other contraindication, the litter may be brought to the side of the bed and level with it and held there, while the patient is directed to roll over onto the bed.   If a third man is available, as he usually is in hospitals, the litter may be *halted* and *lowered* at the side of the bed when, after the patient is lifted, the litter is drawn out by the third bearer, the other two stepping forward and lowering the patient upon the bed.

39. From *litter* to *litter* is executed in the same manner as from *litter* to *bed*.

The movements described may seem rather complicated.   No difficulty presents itself with trained men, however, and in case of accident if 2 or 4 such men are present the comfort and safety of the patient will be assured by following the drill regulations exactly.   Of course, it will be easy for such men to determine what numbers each will take.   If but one trained man is available, no easy problem is presented, but he should take charge of the transportation of the patient best making himself No. 2, and should pick out the other men required from the more intelligent of the willing bystanders.   To each of his assistants he should explain clearly what he wishes done.   Before attempting to lift the patient he should also repeat the necessary commands for doing so and for transfer to the litter until they are thoroughly understood.   He should be especially careful to warn his helpers not to make any change in movement until he directs.   Once the patient is on the litter it will be best to pause for a moment till the necessary explanations in reference to lifting and carrying the litter have been given. This should also be done before ascending stairs or before any movement which involves a decided change in duties. In a word, make haste slowly and prepare for each stage before attempting it.

It will not be necessary for an intelligent man to have more than one experience in hit-and-miss methods for carrying a patient by a number of bearers with pulling here and hauling there, all attended with suffering, to realize, in order to obtain satisfactory results, that cut-and-dried rules must be strictly observed.

The methods followed in loading a patient on an improvised litter should be exactly the same as those which have already been described, nor in carrying the improvised litter will it be desirable to make any changes. When possible, two bearers should generally be used instead of four, as it is so much easier for two men to adapt their movements to each other than it is for four. For the same reason it is best never to employ more than four bearers at one time. When more are desired they should generally be used in relays. With certain improvised litters, however, it will often be wise to have a 5th man appointed to watch the litter so as to warn the bearers if he sees that it is about to come apart. Blankets or rugs employed in place of litters (not blanket litters) are generally carried with more comfort to the patient by four instead of two men and with heavy mattresses, or the like, it is not improbable that it will be necessary to depart from the rule of using but four bearers at the same time.

Not infrequently it proves necessary to transport a patient on a litter in an ordinary wagon or in an ambulance. If the former is used the bottom should always be deeply covered with hay or straw in order to reduce the jolting. Loading and unloading a wagon or ambulance, while not difficult procedures, also require that the bearers act in unison. The following method is recommended. It is adapted from that given in the Hospital Corps Drill Regulations of our army.

To Load the Ambulance or Wagon.

The litter being lifted, is marched to the rear of the ambulance or wagon and wheeled about so that the head of the patient is toward the vehicle and one pace from the step of the ambulance, or the rear of the wagon, as the case may be. The litter is then halted and lowered and the command given:

1. *At sides of litter*, 2. **Posts.**

At posts Nos. 1 and 2 take positions on the right and left, mid-length of the litter, facing it.

1. *Prepare to load*, 2. **Load.**

At the first command the bearers stoop and each grasps a pole firmly with both hands.

At load, the litter is lifted in until a quarter of its length rests upon the floor of the ambulance or wagon and then pushed in.

If the patient is heavy and the bearers are light, the litter is only raised high enough to rest the handles on the floor of the ambulance or wagon; No. 1 then shifts his hands along the pole until he reaches his handles which he supports, while No. 2 gets into the wagon or ambulance, and together they pull and push the litter into place. In case the litter used has stirrups or legs, they must be cleared.

To unload a wagon or ambulance, No. 2 takes position at right rear wheel, and No. 1 at the left rear wheel. The command is:

1. *Prepare to unload*, 2. **Unload.**

At the first command each bearer grasps the handle nearest him. At unload, the bearers partly withdraw the litter, then

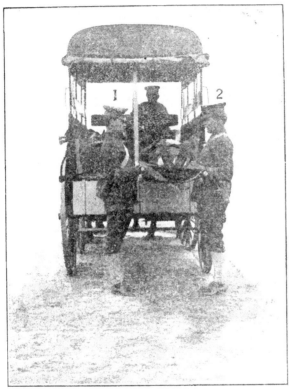

FIG. 65.—Loading ambulance. First movement.
(Drill Regulations, H. C., U. S. A.)

shifting their hands to their respective poles and facing each other, they continue to withdraw it until three-fourths of the length is out, when they lift and lower it to the ground one pace in rear of the vehicle.

It is understood that if the wagon or ambulance is provided with a tail gate that this should be opened and closed as required.

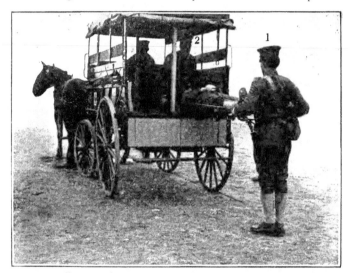

FIG. 66.—Loading ambulance. Second movement.
(*Drill Regulations, H.C., U.S.A.*)

In loading or unloading a litter on a baggage car, the methods described for loading and unloading ambulances and wagons should be adopted.

Straw or hay on which to put the litter should, when possible, be spread on the floor of the baggage car. In a passenger car, so far as the steps are concerned, pursue the methods for ascending and descending stairs. The litter must, of course, be wheeled on the platform. When a passenger car is the last car on a train it may be loaded from the rear like the wagon or ambulance. In a passenger car the litter should be rested on the back of two seats.

Transportation of patients from mines or the hold of a ship sometimes necessitates the vertical instead of the horizontal position of the litter. In this case the patient should first be firmly strapped or tied to the litter. The end of the litter where the patient's head rests should then be raised, by two bearers, one on each side, No. 1 on right, No. 2 on left. The command should be: 1. Prepare to lift end of Litter; 2. Lift. At the command. 1. Prepare to rest end of Litter; 2. Rest. The litter should be allowed to lean against a beam or some other firm object.

The two bearers may then go above No. 1 to seize the right handle, and No. 2 the left. The command should then be: 1. Prepare to Hoist. 2. Hoist.

The litter should be pulled up until the two bearers hold it in the middle, one on each side. At the command: 1. Lower. 2. Litter, they lower it to the ground.

Four bearers can perform this movement much better than two. The command should then be: 1. Additional Squad. 2. Litter. 3. Posts. At the command: 1. Prepare to Hoist. 2. Hoist; the litter in the vertical poistion is gently raised till the two bearers at the top hold it at the middle. It is then lowered to the ground at the command 1. Lower 2. Litter.

Persons slightly injured in the upper part of the body and sick persons who are not very weak or faint may be transported in the sitting position. If a chair can be procured it is generally best to employ it for this purpose. Any strong, light chair will answer, though the ordinary cane-seated arm-chair is handled most easily by bearers. Just as with the litter, transportation in a chair is nat-

14

urally divided into three stages—loading, carrying and unloading. A patient lying down may be lifted into the erect position by one bearer, in the way which will be described in a moment for carrying the patient in the arms, and may then be seated in the chair. The chair may be pushed into the proper position by another person or the bearer may support the patient to the chair. Two bearers, one on each side, may by placing their hands in the patient's armpits, lift him into a chair; or better, they may put the patient's arms around their necks, as shown in Fig. 48. A patient who may be carried in the sitting position will, of course, be able to help himself to some extent.

In unloading, the processes described should be reversed. In loading, carrying and unloading by two bearers, it is absolutely necessary that they work together and the most practical means to insure this is to direct their action by word of command. Therefore, as soon as the bearers are in position to lift the patient the one mutually agreed upon should command: 1. Prepare to Lift, 2. Lift, and when ready to place the patient in the chair, 1. Lower, 2. Patient. To raise the loaded chair again command: 1. Prepare to Lift. 2. Lift. To advance; 1. Forward, 2. March, short sliding steps will be taken. Before attempting to go up or down stairs it will be best to Halt, and to 1. Lower, 2. Patient, and for each step to give the command: 1. Ready, 2. Step. To unload the commands will be: 1. Prepare to Lift, 2. Lift, and 1. Lower, 2. Patient.

A patient able to sit up and steady himself by placing his arms around the bearers' necks may be carried by the Four-handed Seat, the children's "Lady's Chair." To form this each bearer should grasp his left wrist in his right hand and the other bearer's right wrist in his left hand with the knuckles uppermost. The bearers then stoop and place the "chair" under the sitting patient who steadies himself by placing his arms around their necks. It is best also to use the necessary commands here in order that the bearers may act in unison.

In our army, besides the methods already described for carrying

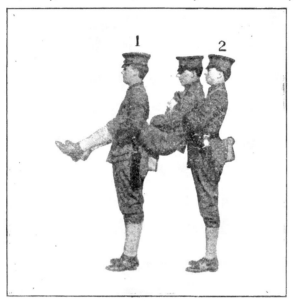

FIG. 67.—Two bearers. Carrying by the extremities.
(*Drill Regulations, H. C., U. S. A.*)

a patient to a litter by two bearers, a method for two bearers called carrying by the extremities is prescribed.

This is performed as follows:

1. *Head and feet.* 2. **Posts.**

At posts, bearers take position at patient, No. 1 between the patient's legs and No. 2 at his head, both facing toward his feet.

1. *Prepare to lift*, 2. **Lift.**

At the first command, the rear bearer having raised the patient to a sitting position, clasps him from behind around the body under the arms, while the front bearer, standing between the legs, passes

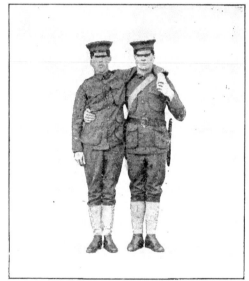

FIG. 68.—One bearer.   Patient raised to erect position.
(*Drill Regulations, H. C., U. S. A.*)

his hands from the outside under the flexed knees.   At lift, both rise together.

This method requires no effort on the part of the patient; but is not applicable to severe injuries of the extremities.

The army methods for transporting a patient by one bearer are as follows:

In the Arms.

The bearer, turning patient on his face, steps astride his body, facing toward the patient's head, and with hands under his armpits lifts him to his knees; then clasping hands over abdomen, lifts him

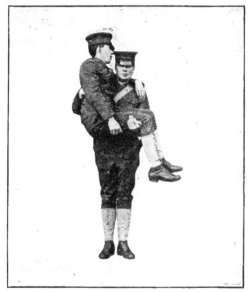

Fig. 69.—One bearer. Patient in the arms.
(*Drill Regulations, H. C., U. S. A.*)

to his feet; he then with his left hand seizes the patient by the left wrist and draws left arm around his (the bearer's) neck and holds it against his left chest, the patient's left side resting against his body, and supports him, with his right arm about the waist.

From this position the bearer with his right arm upon the

patient's back, passes his left under thighs and lifts him into position carrying him well up.

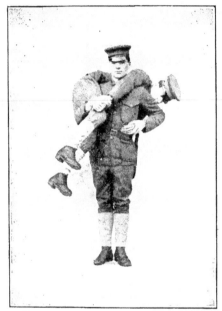

FIG. 70.—One bearer. Patient across back.
(*Drill Regulations, H. C., U. S. A.*)

Across Back.

The patient is first lifted erect as described in previous paragraph, when the bearer with his left hand seizes the right wrist of the patient and draws the arm over his head and down upon his left shoulder, then shifting himself in front, stoops and clasps the right thigh with his right arm passed between the legs, his right hand seizing the patient's right wrist; lastly the bearer with his left hand grasps the patient's left and steadies it against his side, when he rises.

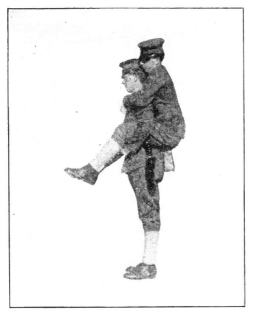

FIG. 71.—One bearer. Patient astride of back.
(*Drill Regulations, H. C., U. S. A.*)

1. *Astride of Back.*

The patient is lifted erect (as described), when the bearer shifts himself to the front of the patient, back to patient, stoops and grasping his thighs, brings him well upon his back.

As the patient must help himself by placing his arms around the bearer's neck, this method is impracticable with an unconscious man.

In lowering the patient from these positions the motions are reversed. Should the patient be wounded in such a manner as to require these motions to be conducted from the right side instead of left, as laid down, the change is simply one of hands—the motions proceed as directed, substituting right for left and *vice versa*.

A patient astride the back of a bearer may, when necessary, be carried up a ladder, though with considerable difficulty. A better method is sometimes used, especially in mines. This requires an apparatus which consists of a wide belt which is held just below the armpits of the bearer by suspenders over the shoulders. From the belt a wide band leads to join the belt on the opposite side. The patient sits in this band supporting himself partially by his hands on the bearer's shoulders.

CHAPTER XI.
ORGANIZATIONS FOR FIRST AID INSTRUCTION.

1. CLASSES. 2. ASSOCIATIONS. 3. RELIEF COLUMNS.

CLASSES.

First Aid classes are now organized in many branches of the Y. M. C. A. and in a number of other associations in various parts of our country.

Such classes should always have a competent doctor as teacher, and it will be found much better not to have more than twenty-five students in a class, as the instructor cannot well supervise the practical work of a greater number.

The material required will be a skeleton and large physiological diagrams showing the arterial and venous systems, the heart and the circulation of the blood, fractures and dislocations. A sufficient number, according to the size of the class, of splints, tourniquets dressings, bandages, etc., should also be provided and one or two litters. When practicable, a boy should be hired as required for anatomical demonstrations.

The course should comprise at least ten sessions, each to last one hour and a half.

It would, of course, be most unwise to try to hamper instructors with directions on how they should teach first aid. It is thought, however, that a few words of advice to instructors to whom the work is new will not be out of place.

Experience has shown that there is a tendency on the part of teachers to pay too much attention to anatomy and physiology at the expense of practical instruction in first aid. Naturally, what should be required of the student is not extensive knowledge of the former subjects, but the ability to treat practically all cases of injury and illness which he may encounter.

Prevention of accidents will be found to be a new subject to most students. The practical value of the instruction depends to a large extent on impressing this subject on all of them:

What has been said above does not mean, of course, that anatomy and physiology are to be neglected. Enough for their purpose should be taught all students of first aid who should also learn the danger of the infection of wounds by germs, bandaging and the transportation of patients, selection being exercised to some extent with the latter subject.

The section Bruises to Fractures and that on Wounds will be found of value to all students, but according to the character and age of his class, the instructor should exercise selection on the weight which he gives to other subjects discussed in this manual. Naturally, the workman must know all about the accidents most common in his particular line of work, and in a class of younger men accidents incident to sports will command more interest and attention.

The Red Cross believes that it accepts a certain responsibility in granting first aid certificates, so this association has determined not to issue such certificates to any but persons who show that they have qualified for them by an examination. This examination is given at the end of any first-aid course by some doctor, other than the teacher, who acts under the instructions of the Red Cross.

Contests between first-aid classes are treated under the proper heading.

ASSOCIATIONS

These organizations have already proved of value in this country, especially in the mining districts of Pennsylvania. The method of organization followed there may be taken as a model. The ratio of first-aid men is estimated as one to sixteen workers and they are so distributed through the mines that one will always be within call in case of accident.

The following which is quoted almost literally from Dr. Shields' First Aid Hand Book gives a very clear description of such associations:

"The association should consist of men of temperate habits, not too young nor too old; men who will not faint at the sight of blood; intelligent, conscientious men, who will expect no compensation but their own inward satisfaction, supplemented, perhaps by gratitude of those whose pains they alleviate.

"Such an association, having first organized temporarily, should then elect a President, Vice-President, Secretary, Treasurer and two or more local physicians as Medical Directors and Lecturers.

"Money will be required for the purchase of First Aid Packets, splints, stretchers, books and other materials. There are several ways by which this can be raised. When the association has been duly organized and the subject of the fund made public, there should be but little difficulty in procuring the funds through some or all of the following channels:

"1. Every man in the mine should contribute a small sum.

"2. The superintendent and other officials of the mine should be asked for a donation. Undoubtedly, they will respond liberally.

"3. The various benefit societies in the town should be approached. A dollar contributed by a benefit society may prevent a raid of a hundred dollars on its treasury.

"4. The members of the association should pay a small entrance fee and monthly dues.

"Regular meetings of the association should be held at least twice a month. The times for lectures and practice can be arranged by the medical directors.

"Each member should be furnished with a First-aid Packet, and the association should always keep a supply in reserve to replace used packets.

"When a member has used his packet he should report at the next meeting, giving full particulars of the kind of accident treated and how the packet was used.

"In factories and mills it will be an easy matter to have the First-aid men evenly distributed. On railroads each association should be so formed as to have at least two First-aid men in each crew. They should always carry their First-aid Packets and reserve supplies in a caboose or baggage car.

"It will be the duty of the medical directors to prescribe a course for the association, extending over a period of eighteen months or two years, at the end of which time they may be examined. To the successful ones should be given certificates of efficiency, then some new members taken into the association.

"Directors should not examine their own association. It will be more satisfactory, for obvious reasons, to have the examinations conducted by directors from sister associations.

"When there are several associations in a town, or vicinity, interest may be kept alive by periodical contests, to consist of stretcher drills, tests of skill in bandaging, and carrying patients, etc. In each contest the winner may be given a badge or boutoniere bearing an appropriate design, and the name, number and location of the association of which the winner is a member. Such will be more highly valued than any other article that gold can buy."

The remarks already made in reference to the teaching of

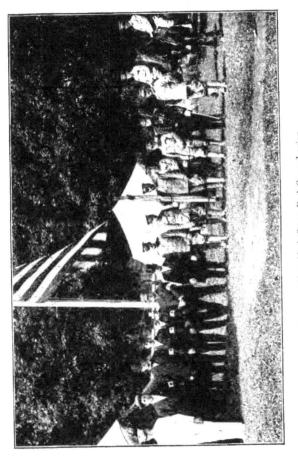

Fig. 72.—New York State Red Cross Legion.

First-aid classes and the material required for such teaching apply equally to the associations which have just been described.

To gain the First-aid Certificate of the Red Cross it is, of course, necessary for students in associations to pass the same examination required from those in classes.

RELIEF COLUMNS.

While the knowledge of First Aid acquired in classes and associations is of great value in diminishing suffering it still lacks something of accomplishing all the good which it might if it were organized. This fact has led to the creation of Relief Columns and Legions by the Red Cross.

A Relief Column is a definite organization of a fixed strength. A number of such columns constitute a Legion.

All individuals in such organizations are compelled to learn First Aid just as are members of classes and associations. The instruction of the former goes somewhat further, however, in order that they may work as a body as well as individually.

The advantages which the Red Cross First-aid organizations possess over individuals instructed in First Aid are the following:

With individuals there is no supervision or control, medical or otherwise, and no organization for combined action which is absolutely necessary for First-aid work on a large scale such as that required in great accidents or in war.

Membership in a relief column compels continuous instruction and practice in First Aid and the care and transportation of sick, wounded and injured. Without this, individuals, however, well taught orginally, cannot keep up their knowledge of the subject.

Certain positions in relief columns afford the best instruction as they require the teaching of other persons. This also permits qualified persons to go much further with their instruction than if they studied First Aid individually.

Relief columns also act as custodians for materials required for First-aid purposes without which it is difficult, if not impossible, to care for sick and injured.

Naturally, too, Relief Columns and Legions as they have the necessary organization may go somewhat further in their good purposes than first aid alone.

For example, the First Legion of the Red Cross which was recently organized in New York State makes the following statement of its objects:

"The objects of this organization shall be the following:

"To give emergency relief to the sick and injured under the direction of physicians or until their services can be procured.

"To provide a volunteer organization of trained men capable of turning out at a moment's notice with all the necessary equipment to render "first aid" to the sick and injured in time of calamity, to transport them and provide for their temporary shelter. Such service, however much needed, shall not be obligatory.

"To prepare a trained body of men to assist the Army Medical Department in time of war and help reduce the terrible and often unnecessary suffering of sick and wounded soldiers, whether on the field, or in camp or hospital. Membership in the Grand Legion does not, however, carry with it any obligation, actual or implied, to give such service; it is entirely voluntary.

"To establish a headquarters where lectures and instruction may be given, drills and exhibitions held, equipment stored and a library and a museum of first-aid appliances be developed.

"To teach ordinary care and forethought for the prevention

of accidents, including what should be done in moments of danger and panic.

"To spread a knowledge of hygiene and assist the world-wide struggle against tuberculosis in which the American National Red Cross has engaged.

"To reach and systematically train in first aid and common care all ages of youth and childhood of both sexes; and to do it through their games, plays and toys.

"To advance the Red Cross, national and international, and thus establish a higher regard for human life and keener sense of brotherhood."

The general rules governing such organization are as follows:

FORMATION.

When a sufficient number of persons to form a relief column or detachment have assembled, they will forward an application for permission to do so to the State Branch of the Red Cross. This will be answered by supplying such persons with the regulations, etc., of relief columns. Before the column is recognized all members will be required to sign the enrollment form which will obligate them to perform their duties satisfactorily, to attend the necessary drills, instructions, formations, etc., and to obey the orders of their officers. Service with the army in war will be purely voluntary.

Authority for the formation of a Relief Column Legion will be granted at once to any four relief columns near enough to each other to make it practicable for them to work together.

On recognition of a relief column the officers will be elected by the members of the column concerned. No one not regularly licensed to practice medicine will be eligible for the office of director.

On recognition of a relief column legion the officers and men

15

of the staff will be selected by joint vote of the members of the relief columns composing it. No one not regularly licensed to practice medicine will be eligible for the office of director in chief.

All members of relief columns and legions must be of good moral character and must be physically qualified for the performance of all duties which may be required of them, except that no physical standard will be fixed for supporting members.

ORGANIZATION.

The organization of a Relief Column is as follows:
    1 Director.
    3 Assistant Directors.
    4 Sub-directors, senior grade.
    16 Sub-directors, junior grade.
    64 Men.

Relief Columns are divided into four Relief Detachments, each of which is organized os follows:
    1 Assistant Director (director in one case).
    1 Sub-director, senior grade.
    4 Sub-directors, junior grade.
    16 Men.

Four relief columns constitute a Relief Column Legion and the term Grand Legion of Relief Columns is applied to the organization comprehending all the relief columns.

Besides the four relief columns mentioned, a Relief Column Legion has the following officers and men:
    1 Director-in-chief.
    2 Assistant Directors (secretaries).
    1 Assistant Director (in charge of stores).
    4 Sub-directors, senior grade.
    4 Men.

DUTIES.

Director-in-chief:

This officer will have general charge of the instruction, discipline and performance of duty of the relief columns as a whole. He will satisfy himself by frequent inspections that each relief column is maintained in a high state of efficiency. He will be held responsible for the stores pertaining to a legion as a whole, and will inspect those of the individual relief columns whenever, in his judgment, this is necessary.

The two assistant directors (secretaries) will assist the director-in-chief in the performance of all duties not connected with supplies, such as drill, discipline, performance of active duty and correspondence.

The assistant director in charge of stores will assist the director-in-chief in all matters pertaining to supplies and will himself be in charge of supplies belonging to the legion as a whole.

The sub-directors and men will assist the above-named officers in the performance of their duties.

The director will command his relief column and will take charge of its instruction, drill and performance of active duty. He will also be held responsible for all property belonging to his column.

The assistant directors will assist the director in the performance of his duties. When the relief detachments act independently, each assistant director will command his own detachment and will be responsible for its property.

The sub-directors, senior grade, correspond to the sergeants 1st class, Hospital Corps, U.S.A., and perform similar duties, assisting in instruction, drill and active service. One is assigned to each detachment. One may properly be placed in direct charge of the supplies belonging to the column with such assistance from subordinate officers and men as is required. When the column

15

operates in detachments, a sub-director, senior grade, will be placed in direct charge of the supplies of the detachment with assistants as prescribed for the column.

The sub-directors, junior grade, are allowed in the proportion of four to each detachment. They perform the duties of sergeants of the Hospital Corps.

The men give first aid and act as litter bearers under the direction of their officers. Their drill and instructions are practiced so as to enable them to do so in a satisfactory manner.

INSTRUCTION.

First aid, and for the present as a tentative scheme of instruction, the Drill Regulations and Outlines of First Aid for the Hospital Corps, United States Army, Revised, 1908. (Selected paragraphs.)

Also special instruction to qualify members for work as an organization.

In teaching, instructors will be expected to explain first-aid work so fully that their classes will understand what they are taught and enough anatomy and physiology will be introduced to enable them to do so. In all cases it will be found necessary to check overzealousness on the part of members of relief columns. They must be made to understand clearly that their part in the treatment of sick, injured and wounded is confined strictly to first aid and to go further than this, except under conditions when it is absolutely impossible to obtain the services of a physician, is not justifiable. Indoor instruction will be divided into twelve periods of two hours each. One-half of the time will be devoted to theoretical and the other half to practical work.

EQUIPMENT.

Naturally, it will not be possible in all cases for relief columns when they are first organized to obtain all the equipment which they will need.

Minimum.—Each two men: One litter (army), One Hospital Corps pouch (army), One canteen (army).

In addition, each column should have enough first-aid packets (instruction), splints and bandages so that each man may have the opportunity to practice their use and application. Fifty instruction first-aid packets, twenty-five assorted-splints and one hundred assorted roller bandages should be procured for this purpose by each relief column. To this should be added a skeleton and the necessary diagrams for instruction.

Each relief column should preferably be a complete unit in itself, with all equipment; but when columns are organized into legions, the latter may properly take in their charge the elaborate equipment for relief stations and the tents and ambulances

UNIFORM.

Two classes of uniform are required to outfit relief columns completely. In the event that only one is procured, preference should be given to the field uniform. The uniforms are similar to the blue (dress) and khaki (field) of the United States Army.

In order to distinguish the Red Cross personnel, their uniform will differ from that of the army in the following particulars:

A cap will be worn with both uniforms. The cap will have an enameled red cross instead of the coat-of-arms. This cross will also appear on the belt plate.

A large Red Cross brassard will be worn on the left arm of each member of the Red Cross personnel.

Sub-directors will wear an enameled red cross on the collar of the blouse on each side of the opening. Sub-directors, junior grade, as a mark or rank, wear on each sleeve of the blouse, three inches above the lower end of the sleeve, a circular red cord. Sub-directors, senior grade, have two such stripes on each sleeve.

Directors-in-chief, directors and assistant directors will have a red cross on the shoulder strap. The director-in-chief will have three parallel stripes of white cord placed vertically on the collar at each side of the collar opening; directors, two such stripes, and assistant directors, one.

FIELD OF ACTIVITIES FOR RELIEF COLUMNS.

Relief columns find an important field for their activities both in peace and in war.

(a) In peace:

(1) Instruction of their personnel in their duties. This will consist not only of indoor teaching, but also of practical field-work at maneuvers and on similar occasions.

(2) Collection of litters, splints, bandages and other material which is essential for the proper performance of such duties.

(3) Active participation in the relief work necessitated by great calamities, disasters, general epidemics, and incident to great public gatherings. Naturally, the methods pursued in accomplishing such work must depend upon circumstances. In general, sick and injured will be succored wherever their illness or injury occurs and will be taken thence to a relief station where further attention will be given them if it is required, with possibly later their final and definite disposition, so far as the relief column is concerned. At large public gatherings, such as great parades and on like occasions, it will generally be found best to post litter squads at convenient points so that they may go promptly to the aid of any one requiring it. Another part of the personnel should establish a relief station at some central point to which patients may be carried for more elaborate treatment or for rest and shelter only. When the services of the entire personnel of a relief column is required for work outside the relief station or under certain other circumstances which readily suggest themselves, the work of the relief station may be entrusted to a "Nursing Detachment."

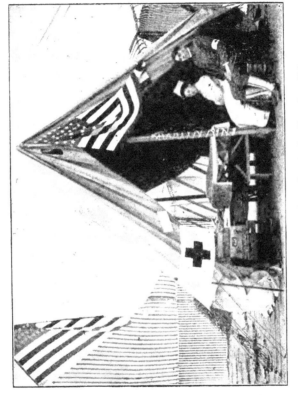

FIG. 73.—Relief Station, Naval Parade, San Francisco, Cal.

Tents or unoccupied stores or houses will be found most suitable for relief stations.

(b) In war:

Generally, relief columns operate as independent units having complete autonomy and only being held responsible to higher authority, like other army units. In war they work under the general direction of the army medical department.

(1) At home:

Service of the character already described for peace between railway stations or ports, and hospitals. In connection with such service, relief stations will sometimes be established by part of the personnel.

(2) In the field: Like services in the lines of communication and sometimes at the actual front.

The by-laws of the New York State Legion of the Red Cross are as follows:

I.

ADMINISTRATION.

The administration of the affairs of this organization shall be vested in a Director and a Board of Administrative Affairs, both subject to the authority of the New York State Branch of the American National Red Cross.

II.

DIRECTOR OF LEGION.

The Director of Legion shall be elected annually by the Legion at the annual meeting.

III.

DUTIES OF DIRECTOR OF LEGION.

The Director of Legion shall be in sole command of the Legion in all matters pertaining to instruction, drill, discipline and the performance of duty, as provided in the regulations of the New York State Branch of the American National Red Cross; and he shall be responsible therefor.

IV.

OTHER OFFICERS OF LEGION.

The three Assistant Directors of Legion, two of whom shall act as secretaries to the Director and one of whom shall be in charge of the stores and be held responsible for all the equipment of the Legion and its condition; and the four subdirectors of senior grade shall all be elected in annual ballot by the Legion.

The officers of each relief column shall similarly be elected by each column in annual ballot, except that subdirectors of junior grade may be appointed by the Director if he shall so be empowered by the column.

V.

BOARD OF ADMINISTRATIVE AFFAIRS.

The Board of Administrative Affairs shall consist of twelve persons, members of this organization, four of whom shall be elected at the annual meeting to serve for three years, in accordance with the rules and regulations as hereinafter set forth.

In constituting the first board, however, there shall be four members elected for three years, four for two years, and four for one year.   In addition, the Director of the Legion shall be a member ex-officio of the Board.

VI.

DUTIES OF BOARD OF ADMINISTRATIVE AFFAIRS.

The duty of the Board of Administrative Affairs shall include the exercise of all powers not conferred on the Director by authority of the New York State Branch of the American National Red Cross. Specifically the Board shall administer the finances of the Legion; provide for audit; devise and carry out plans for filling the quota of the Legion, and increasing its honorary membership; devise and carry out plans for the instruction of junior columns, helpers and other children, when such instruction shall not conflict with the duties of members of the Legion and the authority of the Director; provide entertainments and take such other appropriate action as may promote the interests of the organization.

VII.

OFFICERS OF BOARD.

The officers of the Board shall be: A President, Vice President, Recording Secretary, Corresponding Secretary and Treasurer to serve for a term of one year, or until their successors are elected. The Director of the Legion shall not serve as an officer of the Board.

VIII.

DUTIES OF OFFICERS OF BOARD.

It shall be the duty of the President to preside at all meetings of the Board and to appoint all Committees.

The Vice President shall, in the absence of the President, perform all the duties of the President.

The Recording Secretary shall keep a correct record of the meeting of the Board.

IX.

STANDING COMMITTEES OF BOARD.

The President shall appoint at the annual meeting three members upon the following standing committees: Finance, Auditing, Membership, Entertainment, Press, Junior, Children and Athletics.

X.

Five members of the Board shall constitute a quorum for the transaction of business affairs.

XI.

MEETINGS.

Regular meetings of the Board shall be held on the first Wednesday of each and every month, except July and August.

XII.

SPECIAL MEETINGS.

Special meetings of the Board may be called by the President, at the written request of five members, but such notice of special meeting shall be mailed to each and every member of the Board by the Corresponding Secretary, at least three days before such meeting.

XIII.

MEMBERSHIP.

Membership in this organization shall consist of supporting and active.

1. Supporting members shall consist of those persons who subscribe $2.00 per annum or more.

2. Active members shall consist of those persons who sign the Constitution and By-Laws of the organization and perform the duties of active members as hereinafter provided for.

XIV.

DUES.

The dues of active members shall be $6.00, payable quarterly in advance.

Members in arrears of dues may not vote at the annual meeting.
Members in arrears six months are not in good standing.

XV.

RELIEF COLUMNS.

Each relief column shall elect its own officers in a manner similar to that provided for the election of officers of the Legion. It shall, if unattached to a Legion, elect also a Board of Administrative Affairs whose relation to the Director of Column shall be the same as that of the Board of Administrative Affairs in the Legion is to the Director of Legion.

XVI.

RELIEF SERVICE.

When occasion for service or public demonstration has been foreseen and due notice given to the members of the Legion, then such members, at a regular or special meeting, shall determine whether they desire to give such service as a Legion. Whenever due notice cannot be given, the Director shall be the sole judge of the emergency of the need. Due notice shall be deemed a week's time.

XVII.

ORDER OF BUSINESS.

Roll.
Reading of Minutes.
Application for membership.
Reports of Committees.
Communications.
Unfinished Business.
New Business.
Adjournment.

CHAPTER XI.
FIRST-AID CONTESTS.

Contests between different classes, associations or columns have been found to be one of the best ways to stimulate study of first aid in members of such organizations as well as to arouse public interest in this important subject.

The events in such contests should naturally be those having to do with first-aid problems of special interest to the particular organizations concerned.

Army contests which will generally prove valuable and interesting are the following:

1. Litter bearer contest.—For squads of two; No. 2 in charge.

At command, procure litter, run two hundred paces to a designated patient, render first aid for an injury indicated on a diagnosis tag attached to the patient, place him on the litter, carry him to ambulance or wagon, load ambulance, unload ambulance, carry patient on litter to a designated point fifty paces distant and there lower litter.

2. Litter bearer contest.—Single bearer to start at scratch, run fifty yards, and return to scratch with wounded man supposedly having both legs broken and useless. Wounded man to be personated by a soldier weighing not less than one hundred and fifty pounds, with ankles and thighs strapped together.

3. Carrying wounded contest.—Each team to consist of three men. One man will act as patient and lie down one hundred yards from the scratch. The other two will call off, standing in

line at scratch, litter strapped, three yards in rear of centre of squad. At starting signal, No. 2 procures litter moving at any gait. Squad will then proceed to patient, will open litter, and place patient on it returning to scratch.

If the patient falls off the litter, or squad lets go of one or more handles while patient is on litter the team will be disqualified.

Team will be timed from starting until feet of patient on litter cross the scratch.

4. Hospital Corps contest.—No. 1 has a rifle, No. 2 a rifle and a blanket rolled up. The blanket is on his right shoulder with the ends secured at the left hip by strap or cord. Patient is on ground two hundred yards from scratch. A place is designated as dressing station.

Proceed to patient as quickly as possible, render first aid for the injury noted on the diagnosis tag attached to patient, prepare "blanket litter," place the patient thereon, carry him to designated dressing station.

5. Single bearer contest.—Bearers in line; a patient for each lying on his back fifty paces distant. Run to patient, dress injury indicated on diagnosis tag, lift him erect and carry him across or astride of back to the place of starting.

Points will be estimated by time, character of dressings, comfort of patient, and precision of execution.

6. Contest for three bearers, one with a saddle horse. Run two hundred yards, leading the horse, to a patient lying on the ground; apply the necessary first-aid dressing to the injury designated on the diagnosis tag attached to the patient; improvise a litter, which is to be attached to the saddle and on which the patient is to be transported lying an his back. Load the patient on this litter and return with the horse at a walk. The improvised litter is to be made from material provided.

The two general contests of the Pennsylvania Coal Company

and the Hillside Coal and Iron Company held in 1906 and 1907 were most successful affairs.

In these contests each team consisted of a captain, four men and the subject on whom the demonstration was made.

The following were the events:

FIRST ANNUAL CONTEST.

Event No. 1.—Man insensible from gas, totally helpless. One man to pick him up, carry him 50 feet to good air, lay him down and perform artificial respiration for one minute.

Event No. 2.—Man injured in lower part of body. Two men to form four-handed seat and carry him fifty feet.

Event No. 3.—Man injured; leg broken. Three men to splint his leg with a mine sprag and some straw or hay; make temporary stretcher out of two mine drills and two coats, and carry fifty feet.

Event No. 4.—Man injured; wound right side of temple; one man to open packet and dress wound.

Event No. 5. General contest of eight teams. Man unconscious; wounds, simple fracture of right arm between elbow and shoulder; crushed foot with severe hemorrhage; apply tourniquet for bleeding, splints for fracture, perform artificial respiration for one minute, place on stretcher, carry fifty feet over car loaded with coal, pile of mine rock, then over fence and place in ambulance.

SECOND ANNUAL CONTEST.

Event No. 1.—One man contest, artificial respiration. Man nsensible from electric shock, lying on the wire. One man to take him off, carry thirty feet and perform artificial respiration.

Event No. 2.—Two men contest, carrying injured man. Simple fracture of left leg, between knee and ankle, conscious. Two men to form four-handed seat and carry fifty feet.

Event No. 3.—Three men contest, temporary stretcher.

Simple fracture of left leg, between knee and ankle. Three men to splint fracture with hay and sprags, make temporary stretcher out of two coats and two drills, carry fifty feet and take off stretcher.

Event No. 4.—One man contest, dressing an injury with first-aid packet. A fracture of bones of nose from a kick, with severe bleeding. Stop bleeding and dress with first-aid packet.

Event No. 5.—General team contest to determine winner of loving cup. Simple fracture of right thigh between the hip and knee, left collar bone broken and scalp wound on top of head; compound fracture of left arm between wrist and elbow. Dress open wounds with first-aid packet, splint fracture, place on stretcher, carry over fence, car, pile of rock, and put in ambulance.

The prizes offered in the first four events were framed, hand- · engrossed certificates which were given to the successful contestants. In the fifth event the first prize was a loving cup, the second $25 in gold, and the third a certificate to the team. All of the prizes, except one, were presented by the companies.

Appropriate contests for Relief Columns and Legions besides those mentioned above are such as will show the relative ability of such bodies as organizations.

An excellent event of this character is to have the columns assemble and procure necessary supplies then to march to a designation point, leave a part of the organization there to establish a relief station sending the other part to bring in subjects tagged with diagnosis tags giving the injury in each case. Speed and execution each to count equally in determining winner.

An officer in charge, judges, a time-keeper and a starter will of course be required for any of these contests.

16

REFERENCES.

Accidents and Emergencies, Dulles.
Ambulance Hand-Book, St. Andrew's Ambulance Association.
A Nos Soldats, Soins et Conseils par le Docteur A. Tissot.
Barton First Aid Text-Book.
Boys' Drill Regulations of the National First Aid Association of
 . America.
Care of the Feet, Pepoon, Nurses' Journal of the Pacific Coast.
Diseases of the Skin. Stelwagon.
Drill Regulations and Outlines of First Aid for the Hospital Corps,
 United States Army, 1908.
Emergencies, Bailey.
First Aid in Accidents, Dickson.
First Aid in Illness and Injury, Pilcher.
First Aid Hand-Book, Shields.
First Aid Manuals, Service, and Stretcher Bearer Drill Books, various,
 including Austrian, British, French, German, Japanese, etc.
First Aid to the Injured and Management of the Sick, Lawless.
First Aid to the Injured and Sick Warwick and Tunstall.
First Aid to the Injured in Coal Mines, Shields.
First Aid to the Injured, Esmarch.
First Aid to the Injured, St. John's Ambulance Association.
First Aid Principles, St. John's Ambulance Association.
First Aid Text-Book, American National Red Cross.
Hand-Book of First Aid to the Injured by Bowditch Morton, M.D.,
 revised by Ellworth Eliot, M. D., and Louis Faugeres Bishop,
 M. D.
Home Nursing and Hygiene, Hand-Book, St. Andrew's Ambulance
 Association.
Manual des Premiers Secours a l'usage des Sous-Officers et Soldats.
Manual of First Aid, Austin.

Pamphlets, St. John's Ambulance Association.
Pamphlets, St. John's Ambulance Brigade.
Practical First Aid, Robertson.
Principles and Practice of Medicine, Osler.
Prompt Aid to the Injured, Doty.
Quelques Conferences pour l'instruction des Infirmiers Regimentaires par M. Cros, Medicin-Major, de 2me Classe.
Relief Corps Regulations, New York State Branch, American National Red Cross.

INDEX.

241

9 789354 445781